Major Histocompatibility System

Major Histocompatibility System

THE GORER SYMPOSIUM

EDITED BY

SIR PETER MEDAWAR

OM, CH, CBE, FRS

AND

T. LEHNER

MD, FRCPath

BLACKWELL SCIENTIFIC PUBLICATIONS

OXFORD LONDON EDINBURGH

BOSTON PALO ALTO MELBOURNE

© 1985 by
Blackwell Scientific Publications
Editorial offices:
Osney Mead, Oxford, OX2 0EL
8 John Street, London, WC1N 2ES
23 Ainslie Place Edinburgh, EH3 6AJ
52 Beacon Street, Boston
    Massachusetts 02108, USA
744 Cowper Street, Palo Alto
    California 94301, USA
107 Barry Street, Carlton
    Victoria 3053, Australia

First published 1985

Set by Eta Services (Typesetters) Ltd,
Beccles, Suffolk
and printed and bound
in Great Britain at
the Alden Press, Oxford

DISTRIBUTORS

USA
    Blackwell Mosby Book Distributors
    11830 Westline Industrial Drive
    St Louis, Missouri 63141

Canada
    Blackwell Mosby Book Distributors
    120 Melford Drive, Scarborough
    Ontario M1B 2X4

Australia
    Blackwell Scientific Book Distributors
    31 Advantage Road, Highett
    Victoria 3190

British Library
Cataloguing in Publication Data

Major histocompatibility system,
    1. Histocompatibility
    2. Immune response
    I. Medawar, P.B.   II. Lehner, T.
    616.07'95   QR184.3

ISBN 0-632-01358-3

Contents

Preface

Peter A. Gorer embarked on the work which led to the discovery of the H-2 major histocompatibility system of mice about 50 years ago. The significance of this discovery has surpassed his initial expectation of producing immunity to tumours, for as we now know, the major histocompatibility system is involved in the recognition of self as opposed to non-self and in the regulation of the immune response. It is particularly sad that Peter Gorer did not live long enough to enjoy the development of his basic concept of the major histocompatibility system.

The British Society for Immunology wished to honour the outstanding contribution Peter Gorer made to the science of immunology by dedicating this symposium to his memory. The scientific committee consisting of Dr Brigitte Askonas, Dr Walter Bodmer and the Editors were anxious to invite contributions from key authorities in the field of immunogenetics. The symposium took place on 10 November 1983 in London, under the auspices of the British Society for Immunology. The scientific content is published in this volume, and it is hoped that this will also mark a historical occasion of a fundamental discovery in immunology.

We wish to acknowledge the support we have received, particularly during the initiation of this symposium, from Drs Gordon Ada, Brigitte Askonas, Baruj Benacerraf, Walter Bodmer, Sir McFarlane Burnet, John Humphrey, Jean Dausset, Rodney Porter, George Snell and Jack Strominger. We thank the Committee of the British Society for Immunology for making this symposium possible. We gratefully acknowledge the assistance we received from Peter Gorer's friends and colleagues at Guy's Hospital Medical School, where he carried out much of the research. We particularly wish to thank Drs Sidney Cohen, George Houston, Charles Joiner, Maurice Lessof and Mr Donald Bompas, and for the financial support for the Peter Gorer Lecturership received from the Governors of Guy's Hospital Medical School.

Sir Peter Medawar
Thomas Lehner

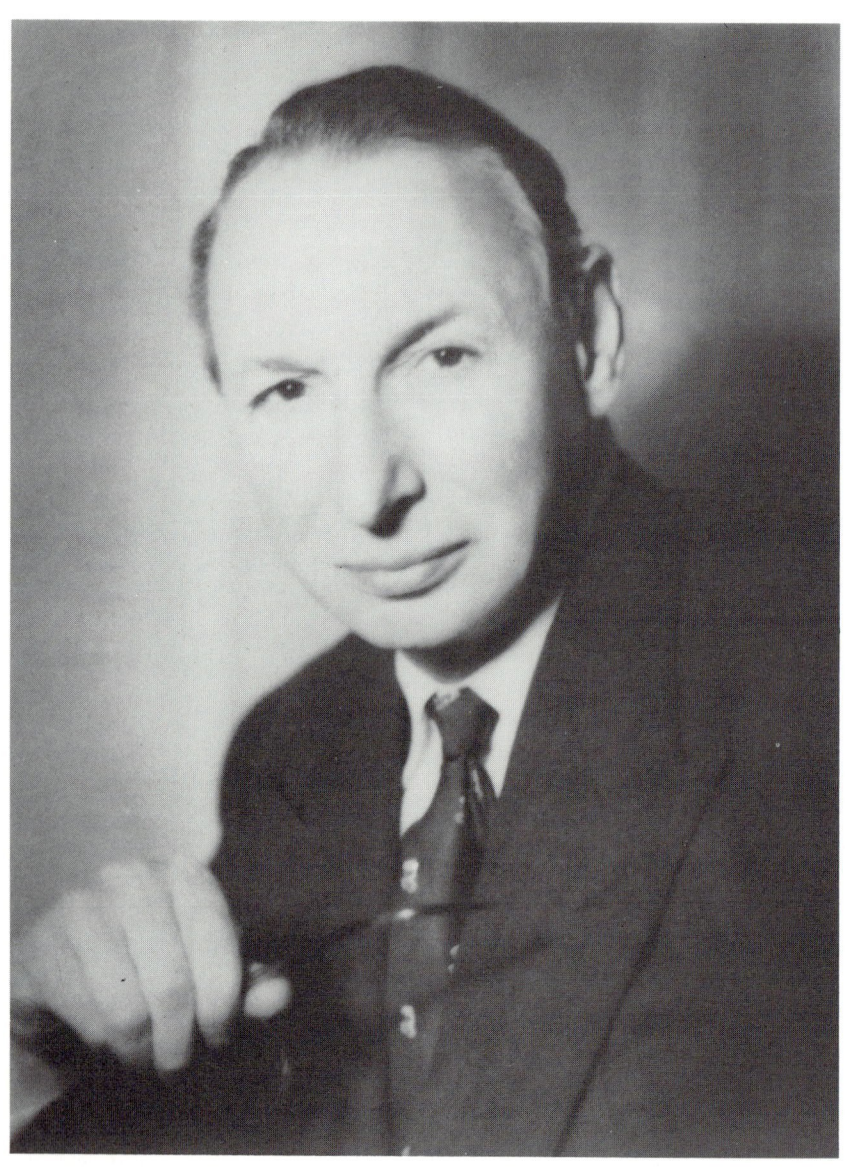

Fig. 1.1. P. A. Gorer (1907–1961).

Chapter 1
The work of Peter Alfred Gorer

Sir Peter Medawar

Peter Gorer died in 1961 at the height of his scientific powers having made a number of very important discoveries, the developments of which are the subject of this conference. Had he been spared, he would at this meeting have been only 76—not a great feat of longevity nowadays—and Gorer indeed was quite a bit younger than that other great figure in the immunogenetics of transplantation: George Snell.

University College London

When Gorer graduated in medicine in 1932 he had the good judgement to apply to study under J. B. S. Haldane in University College London. University College is the oldest and largest of the colleges that together make up the rather ramshackle federation known as London University. It has played—is still playing—a very important part in transplantation biology. Indeed, it is not going too far to say that transplantation biology itself was the gift to the world of University College London.

Haldane turned Gorer's thoughts to the idea of looking for antigenic variation in mice, a project made feasible by the fact that at the time Dr Hans Gruneberg, a sacerdotal figure in mouse genetics, was also in University College.

Gorer's first discovery was that in a normal human serum, his own, he could distinguish two or possibly three kinds of red cells in mice: his serum agglutinated the red cells of A-strain mice strongly, of CBA strain feebly and of C57 mice not at all. The results of some simple crosses suggested that the property of being agglutinable by Gorer's serum behaved as a straightforward Mendelian dominant. For his own serum Gorer soon substituted an antiserum made in the conventional way, by the deliberate injection of mouse erythrocytes into rabbits. Three antigens could now be recognized. Antigen I was shared by A and CBA; antigen II was represented strongly in A and weakly in CBA; antigen III was recognized in all three strains. Antigen II was clearly of special importance and Gorer turned now to studying its relevance to the transplantability of a sarcoma that had arisen 'spontaneously' in an

A-strain mouse. This tumour would grow only in mice that had an A-strain parent: it grew in A mice and in the progeny of hybrids between A-strain and other strains, but would not grow in C57 at all.

Histocompatibility-2

Results of this general kind had already been observed and reported upon by immunogeneticists in the Jackson Laboratory in Bar Harbor, Maine, by men such as Snell, Tyzzer, Bittner and the Director, Clarence Little. But Peter Gorer introduced a novel twist into the interpretation of the results. The Bar Harbor workers and others had spoken of Mendelian factors, the possession of which conferred *susceptibility* to the growth of strain-specific tumours. Gorer saw that, although susceptibility and resistance were simply the opposite sides of the same coin, it would make more sense in the context of general immunology if the possession by the tumour of antigen II was said to excite *resistance* in mice that lacked it, and he formulated very precisely the immunological interpretation of the acceptance or rejection of tumour transplants. Gorer thought in terms of alloantigens: he was not inclined to credit the notion that tumours might have distinctive antigenic properties simply by reason of being tumours (as Foley was later on to show they did). His interpretation was confirmed by a demonstration that tumours containing antigen II would arouse specific antibodies in mice that lacked it. On the serological side, certain complications had arisen that were attributed to variations of 'avidity' and these complexities can be seen now to portend the complexities of histocompatibility locus H-2, as Gorer and Snell in friendly collusion agreed to call it.

H-2, the major histocompatibility complex of mice, was clearly a complex locus that put Gorer in mind of the rhesus system in man. Antibodies were often difficult to demonstrate. Gorer would not have them referred to or even thought of as 'incomplete antibodies'. They were to be thought of merely as 'inconvenient' antibodies. Indeed, a demonstration of these antibodies in haemagglutination *in vitro* called for the use of dextran and absorbed human AB serum, and the whole recipe put one irresistibly in mind of passages from *Macbeth*, Act IV, Scene I; nevertheless, as those who know him could have predicted, my colleague Leslie Brent made the technique work reliably and reproducibly. This is a good moment to say how much Peter Gorer owed to the skill and sense of participation of his exceptionally able technicians, Maureen Tuffrey and Barbara Mikulska.

The old and the new University College teams

Peter Gorer left University College for the Lister Institute before joining the Department of Pathology in Guy's Hospital. It has been a lasting source of regret to Rupert Billingham, Leslie Brent and myself that we did not overlap with Gorer, but we kept closely in touch with each other and met from time to time at dinner together in Simpson's Restaurant in the Strand (then as now the best value for money in London). Peter's team included three brilliant young colleagues, Bernard Amos, Ted Boyse and Richard Batchelor, all of whom made international reputations; their good sense in going to work under Gorer was the equal of Gorer's in apprenticing himself to Jack Haldane after his graduation. However it may have begun, the conversation always managed to work round to the question of what exactly the antibodies *did* in the rejection of transplants. We needled each other in a way that was sometimes especially fruitful. To revenge myself on Gorer for having once suggested to me that I was wasting my time on skin grafts and should turn instead to the use of tumours, I told Peter that no results in transplantation theory could be regarded as valid unless they were shown to be true of skin grafts also: I wanted to know whether skin homografts could excite antibody formation. Peter Gorer and Rupert Billingham resolved to collaborate in answering this question and, of course, found that they do: indeed, they are very good at raising antibodies; but Billingham, Brent and I did a large number of strenuous experiments which showed to our minds conclusively that antibodies themselves are not inimical to the grafts of normal tissue. We were all in favour of cell-mediated immunity, which Peter Gorer never really took to. Indeed, he flunked the DPhil thesis of a former pupil of mine who had had the temerity to discover the modality of immunity which, with characteristic infelicity, we now describe as 'adoptive immunity'. However, in the outcome the candidate did not have to write 'failed DPhil' after his name. He became instead one of the world's principal authorities in immunology generally.

In spite of this difference of opinion, the more of Simpson's excellent house burgundy we drank, the more readily we agreed that both parties were right and that in due course we should discover how cells and antibodies colluded in causing homografts to be destroyed.

Gorer was an educated man who did not conceal the degree to which his sensibilities were constantly outraged by the etymological chamber of horrors that transplantation biology had turned into. He accordingly wrote a paper for a meeting of the Transplantation Society entitled

'Transplantese', which led to the supplanting of 'homografts' and 'hetero-grafts' by 'allografts' and 'xenografts'.

The importance of the MHC

Those who were attracted into transplantation biology by the problem of allograft rejection usually feel that the great importance of the MHC is that it can be used to facilitate the acceptance of grafts in clinical practice: and we must not forget that Gorer framed the conceptual background and devised many of the techniques used in the uncovery and analysis of MHC of man, HLA. On the other hand, those attracted into transplantation biology for immunological and genetic reasons regard its practical usefulness in transplantation as by no means the most interesting or important of its aspects. Let us be clear that the importance of MHC is two-fold:

(i) HLA defines a new system of genetic polymorphism in man that is at least as important as the polymorphism of blood group antigens. As such, it has already made possible the identification of genotypes associated with especially high risks of ankylosing spondylitis, multiple sclerosis and insulin-dependent diabetes. This is important enough and of course the whole story has not yet been told.

(ii) The MHC plays a crucially important part in the recognition of 'self'. Its function was once likened by an American post-doctoral student working in the CRC to a system of signals which empowered every cell in the body to cry out 'It's me! it's me!', later emended by popular request to 'It is I! It is I!'. I do not think the analogy is a very good one anyway. I see it as a better analogy that the MHC has much the function of a carrier wave in radio transmission: this is the wave to which a radio set is tuned and a radio signal is generated by an amplitude, frequency or phase modulation of the carrier wave. The more I think about this aspect of the working of MHC the more important I think it is.

Conclusion

Peter Gorer played a vital part in all of this important work, of which he must be regarded as the conceptual ancestor. Much of the work that is to be described at this symposium can be traced back to sources in Peter Gorer's mind, and I shall entertain myself during this meeting by thinking what a very great delight this symposium would have been to him, and how proud he would be that his brilliant pupils are playing such a leading role in it.

Chapter 2
Structure, regulatory polymorphisms, and allelic hypervariable regions in murine I-A and I-E molecules

H. O. McDevitt, Diane J. Mathis, C. Benoist, L. Mengle-Gaw, Madge R. Kanter & Virginia E. Williams

Department of Medical Microbiology, Stanford University Medical Center, Stanford, California 94305, U.S.A.

Summary. Analysis of mRNA and genomic clones reveals several mechanisms of failure of synthesis of the E_α polypeptide chains. Comparison of predicted amino acid sequences from cDNA sequence of I-A and I-E, α and β chains shows that most allelic variation occurs in the first domain in the 3-4 'allelic hypervariable' regions in A_α, A_β and E_β, while E_α is relatively invariant. This leads to some preliminary prediction about the three-dimensional configurations of Ia molecules.

The genes of the murine major histocompatibility system (MHS) encode at least two classes of cell surface molecules which are intimately involved in cell–cell interaction, antigen presentation by macrophages and recognition of foreign antigens (McDevitt, 1981; Klein *et al.*, 1981). The class I MHS molecules are 44,000 molecular weight (MW) glycoproteins bound in a strong, non-covalent association with β_2 microglobulin (MW 12,000). Class I molecules are expressed on all nucleated cells, and influence the specificity of cytotoxic lymphocytes (CTL). The class II MHS molecules, the murine I region-associated (Ia) antigens, map in the I region of the murine MHS (designated histocompatibility-2 or H-2) and influence the ability of the animal to develop effective helper T cells to T cell-dependent foreign antigens (McDevitt, 1981; Klein *et al.*, 1981). Two categories of Ia molecular complexes have been described in the mouse: the I-A complex, composed of two subunits, A_α (34,000 MW) and A_β (29,000 MW), encoded by genes which map in the I-A subregion; and the I-E complex consisting of E_α (34,000 MW) encoded by a gene mapping in the I-E subregion and E_β (29,000 MW) encoded by a gene which maps in the I-A subregion (Benoist *et al.*, 1983a). The invariant chain, I_i, is found associated with both I-A and I-E molecules, but its structural gene does not map in the MHS, or on the murine 17th chromosome.

Until recently, structural information about Ia antigens has been scanty due to the small amounts of these molecules expressed on B lymphocytes, macrophages (or antigen-presenting cells) and activated T cells, which has made it difficult to obtain sufficient amounts of pure Ia molecules for determination of primary amino acid sequence.

The I-A molecule is expressed on B cells of all mouse H-2 haplotypes. Its human counterpart is the HLA-DC molecule. In contrast, certain H-2 haplotypes fail to express the I-E complex at the cell surface (Jones, Murphy & McDevitt, 1981), unlike its human counterpart, the HLA-DR molecule, which is universally expressed in all individuals studied to date. Mice of the $H-2^b$ and $H-2^s$ haplotypes fail to express the I-E complex, apparently because they do not synthesize E_α, even though normal *un*glycosylated E_β chain is readily detectable in the cytoplasm (Jones *et al.*, 1981). On the other hand, $H-2^q$ and $H-2^f$ haplotype mice do not make detectable amounts of either E_α or E_β (Jones *et al.*, 1981). This lack of an expressed I-E molecule has been correlated with a diminished immune response to several antigens (Jones *et al.*, 1981; Benacerraf & Dorf, 1976; Schwartz *et al.*, 1976; Solinger *et al.*, 1979). Thus, in most strains, mice must express E_α and $E_\alpha:E_\beta$ heterodimer in order to respond to the Glu,Lys,Phe random synthetic polypeptide. Failure to express the I-E complex on the cell surface therefore has very real functional immunological significance.

It has not yet become clear how Ia molecules regulate the immune response at the molecular level. Many investigators agree that one of the major cellular sites of action of class II MHS (Ia) antigens is at the level of the antigen-presenting macrophage (Rosenthal, 1978). It has been postulated that Ia molecules regulate the immune response by interacting directly with foreign antigen on the surface of the macrophage, this protein–protein interaction thereby 'selecting' particular determinants for presentation to the T cell (Rosenthal, 1978). Other investigators have presented evidence arguing that Ia antigens act *in*directly by associating with self antigens in the thymus, leading to self tolerance and altering the repertoire of T cell receptors (Nagy *et al.*, 1981).

If Ia molecules interact with foreign antigens on the macrophage cell surface, it is not known whether this occurs in/on an 'active site' on the Ia molecule, analogous to the antibody combining sites on an antibody molecule. The alternative 'direct interaction' model would postulate contact between Ia molecule and foreign antigen at many different points on the surface of the I-A molecule. The first 'direct interaction' model would predict clustering of functionally important allelic variations in amino acid sequence at an 'active site'. The second model would predict allelic amino acid sequence variations at scattered points on the three-dimensional configuration of the Ia molecule.

To study these questions, we have used the techniques of molecular genetics to determine the primary structure of Ia antigens, some of the mechanisms of regulation of their expression, and the molecular localization of their genetic polymorphisms. Genomic DNA clones for the A_α and E_α polypeptide chains were selected from an A/J (H-2^a) genomic library, utilizing a cDNA clone for the human p34 (HLA-DR$_\alpha$) gene product (Benoist *et al.*, 1983a). cDNA clones encoding A_α and E_α were isolated from cDNA libraries constructed by standard techniques, utilizing a 'single copy' probe obtained from a genomic A_α clone by restriction enzyme digestion (Benoist *et al.*, 1983a). The isolated cDNA clones, and portions of the genomic clones, were sequenced in both directions by standard DNA sequencing techniques (Sanger *et al.*, 1980; Fuhrman *et al.*, 1981; Maxman & Gilbert, 1980). The cDNA sequences were used to deduce the amino acid sequences of E_α and A_α polypeptides.

Comparison with partial sequences of an E_α genomic clone obtained by Das, Lawrence & Weissman (1983) permitted delineation of the intron–exon organization, and a clearer understanding of the organization of the protein domains of the E_α and A_α polypeptides.

Figure 2.1 presents the predicted amino acid sequence for the A_α^k gene product compared with that for the E_α^k gene product. Fifty percent of the residues are identical. In general, there are no long stretches of identity. Rather, identical residues are interspersed between short stretches of non-homology, the most dissimilar regions being the cytoplasmic tails and the leader peptides. The amino termini of the mature, processed, proteins (residues 1–23) are also quite divergent. In contrast, the remainder of the first domain and many parts of the second domain are much more conserved (55% and 60% identity, respectively). The greatest similarity is in the transmembrane region (residues 192–214 in E_α) where 18 of the 23 amino acids are identical.

The most interesting result of this comparison is the extensive homology between E_α and A_α. It seems clear that E_α and A_α have similar if not identical functions, since each participates as the 'heavy chain' in an Ia molecular complex expressed on the cell surface, and I-A and I-E molecules both function in regulating antigen-specific immune responses (McDevitt, 1981; Klein *et al.*, 1981; Jones *et al.*, 1981; Benacerraf & Dorf, 1976; Schwartz *et al.*, 1976; Solinger *et al.*, 1979). However, only the amino termini and the cytoplasmic domains show no homology between these two α chains. In haplotypes such as H-2^b and H-2^s (which express E_β but not

Domain labels: I.P.   D1   D2   TC

```
Aα  ....Pro Gly Gly Leu Cys Ser Arg Ala Leu Ile Leu Gly Val Leu Ala Leu Thr Thr Met Leu Ser Leu Cys Gly Gly
Eα  NH2-Met Ala Thr Ile Gly Ala Leu Val Leu Gly Phe Phe Ile Ala Val Leu Met Ser Gln Lys Ser Trp Ala
                                                                                                        1

Aα  Glu Asp Asp Ile Glu Ala Asp His Val Gly Ser Tyr Gly Ile Thr Val Tyr Gln Ser Pro Gly Asp Ile Gly Gln Tyr
Eα  Ile Lys Glu Glu His Thr Ile Ile Gln Ala Glu Phe Tyr. Leu Leu Pro Asp Lys Arg Gly Glu Phe
                                                                                                        10

Aα  Thr Phe Glu Phe Asp Gly Asp Glu Leu Phe Tyr Val Asp Leu Asp Lys Lys Glu Thr Val Trp Met Leu Pro Glu Phe
Eα  Met Phe Asp Phe Asp Gly Asp Glu Ile Phe His Val Asp Ile Glu Lys Ser Glu Thr Ile Trp Arg Leu Glu Glu Phe
        23                                                                   36

Aα  Ala Gln Leu Arg Arg Phe Glu Pro Gln Gly Gly Leu Gln Asn Ile Ala Thr Gly Lys His Asn Leu Glu Ile Leu Thr
Eα  Ala Lys Phe Ala Ser Phe Glu Ala Gln Gly Ala Leu Ala Asn Ile Ala Val Asp Lys Ala Asn Leu Asp Val Met Lys
        49                                                                   62

Aα  Lys Arg Ser [Asn Ser Thr] Pro Ala Thr Asn
Eα  Glu Arg Ser [Asn Asn Thr] Pro Asp Ala Asn
        75                      84

Aα  Glu Ala Pro Gln Ala Thr Val Phe Pro Lys Ser Pro Val Leu Leu Gly Gln Pro Asn Thr Leu Ile Cys Phe Val Asp
Eα  Val Ala Pro Glu Val Thr Val Leu Ser Arg Ser Pro Val Asn Leu Gly Glu Pro Asn Ile Leu Ile Cys Phe Ile Asp
        85                                                                   98

Aα  Asn Ile Phe Pro Pro Val Ile [Asn Ile Thr] Trp Leu Arg Asn Ser Lys Ser Val Thr Asp Gly Val Tyr Glu Thr Ser
Eα  Lys Phe Ser Pro Pro Val Val [Asn Val Thr] Trp Leu Arg Asn Gly Arg Pro Val Thr Glu Gly Val Ser Glu Thr Val
        111                                                                  124

Aα  Phe Phe Val Asn Arg Asp Tyr Ser Phe His Lys Leu Ser Tyr Leu Thr Phe Ile Pro Ser Asp Asp Asp Ile Tyr Asp
Eα  Phe Leu Pro Arg Asp Asp His Leu Phe Arg Lys Phe His Tyr Leu Pro Phe Leu Pro Ser Thr Asp Asp Phe Tyr Asp
        137                                                                  150

Aα  *Cys Lys Val Glu His Trp Gly Leu Glu Glu Pro Val Leu Lys His Trp
Eα   Cys Glu Val Asp His Trp Gly Leu Asp Glu Pro Leu Arg Lys His Trp
         163                                      176

Aα  Glu Pro Glu Ile Pro Ala Pro Met Ser Glu Leu Thr Glu Thr Val Val Cys Ala Leu Gly Leu Ser Val Gly Leu Val
Eα  Glu Phe Glu Glu Lys Thr Leu Leu Pro Glu Thr Lys Glu Asn Val Val Cys Ala Leu Gly Leu Phe Val Gly Leu Val
        179                                                                  192

Aα  Gly Ile Val Val Gly Thr Ile Phe Ile Ile Gln Gly Leu Arg Ser Gly Gly Thr Ser Arg His Pro Gly Pro Leu-COOH
Eα  Gly Ile Val Val Gly Ile Ile Leu Ile Met Lys Gly Ile Lys Lys Arg Asn Val Val Glu Arg Arg Gln Gly Ala Leu-COOH
        205                                                                  218                          230
```

Fig. 2.1. Predicted amino acid sequence of A^k and E^k based on the cDNA clone nucleotide sequences.

E_α), there is no detectable association between E_α and A_α (Jones *et al.*, 1981). Thus, the striking degree of amino acid sequence homology is *not* reflected in a similar ability of A_α to associate with E_β (or, in other haplotypes, of E_α to associate with A_β). This suggests that the short stretches of non-homology in the amino terminal part of domain one, and scattered throughout domain two, are important structural features which serve to give a distinct tertiary structure to A_α and E_α such that they can only associate with their corresponding A_β and E_β 'light chain'.

It is not yet clear whether an organism derives an advantage from having two types of Ia molecules. This may be the case, since the human has *three* types of Ia molecules (DR, DC and SB), with five expressed α chain genes, and as many as seven expressed β chain genes. It is even more puzzling that several mouse strains (carrying the H-2[b,s,f,q] haplotypes) fail to express the I-E complex on the surface of B cells, antigen-presenting cells, or activated T cells. Because of the extensive amino acid sequence homology between murine E_α and HLA-DR p34 (Das *et al.*, 1983) it is striking that the expression of the E_α polypeptide (and therefore the entire I-E molecule) chain is frequently disposed with in the mouse, while p34 is apparently always expressed in man. To study this further, an effort was begun to analyse the possible mechanisms for failure of expression of the E_α gene product in mice bearing the H-2[b,s,f,q] haplotypes. These findings have been presented in detail elsewhere (Mathis *et al.*, 1983a) and will be summarized briefly here.

Figure 2.2 depicts a Northern blot analysis of E_α poly-A($+$) mRNA transcripts in several H-2 congenic mouse strains. Poly-A($+$) RNA was isolated from spleens of MHS congenic mice, electrophoresed in agarose gels, and hybridized with a nick-translated E_α genomic DNA probe. Mice carrying the H-2[k,d,f,u] haplotypes synthesized readily detectable amounts of mRNA. On the other hand, mice carrying the H-2[b,s] haplotypes (B10 and B10.S) synthesized no detectable E_α mRNA. Mice of the H-2[q] haplotype (B10.G) synthesized very low levels of E_α mRNA which are detectable upon examination of the audioradiograph, but are not easy to detect in the printed version of Fig. 2.2.

As mentioned, mice of the H-2[b,s,f,q] haplotypes fail to express E_α and E_β on the cell surface. Results of the Northern analysis shown in Fig. 2.2 indicate that there are, in all likelihood, at least three separate mechanisms for failure of E_α expression. First, H-2[b,s] mice fail to synthesize any detectable mRNA for the E_α gene. Mice of the H-2[q] (B10.G) haplotype synthesize extremely low, but detectable, amounts of a normal sized E_α mRNA. Mice of the H-2[f] (B10.M) haplotype express reduced amounts of

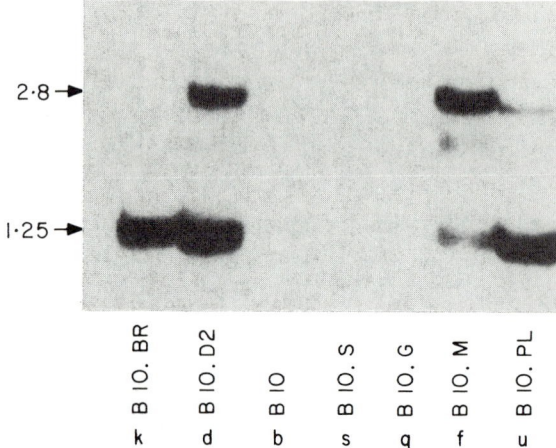

Fig. 2.2. Northern blot analysis of poly-A(+) RNA from the indicated inbred strains, probed with an E_2^k cDNA probe. B10.BR = H.2^k; B10.D2 = H.2^d; B10 = H.2^b; B10.5 = H.2^s; B10.G = H.2^q; B10.M = H.2^f; B10.PL = H.2^u.

a mRNA which appears to be of the normal size (1·3 kb), and quite large amounts of a high molecular weight mRNA which is also present in the H-2^{d,u} (B10.D2 and B10.PL) haplotypes, but is not seen in the H-2^k haplotype (B10.BR).

Systematic analysis of restriction enzyme digests, and double restriction enzyme digests, of an E_α^b genomic clone compared with an E_α^k genomic clone revealed a 600 base pair deletion which spanned the promoter region in the corresponding normally expressed E_α^k genomic clone (Mathis *et al.*, 1983b). It is not yet known what abnormality in transcription or processing of mRNA is responsible for the extremely low amounts of E_α^q mRNA in B10.G mice or the normal amounts of E_α^f mRNA which are present in H-2^f mice (B10.M) which also fail to express any detectable E_α^f polypeptide chain. Experiments are currently in progress to isolate cDNA clones from the H-2^f haplotype to determine the defect(s) in this mRNA which lead to a failure in translation.

Thus, there are three separate mechanisms for failure to express E_α, and therefore the I-E molecule. This is of interest because its human counterpart (DRp34) is always expressed in all individuals studied to date, and because the E_α gene shows nearly complete sequence conservation in the haplotypes in which it is expressed (Mathis *et al.*, 1983b). The structural characteristics of the I-E molecule which permit it to be dispensed with, and the structural features of the corresponding I-A complex which appear to make it necessary for murine survival, are unknown. Clearly, these regulatory polymorphisms can have functional consequences (Jones *et al.*, 1981; Benacerraf & Dorf, 1976; Schwartz *et al.*, 1976; Solinger *et al.*, 1979). However, these functional consequences are not incompatible with survival either in the laboratory or in the wild, since approximately 20% of wild mice lack a detectable I-E molecular complex expressed on the surface of B cells and macrophages (Altman & Katz, 1979; Klein *et al.*, 1976; Duncan, Wakeland & Klein, 1979).

A question of great interest concerns the possible existence on Ia molecules of a 'binding site' for foreign antigens. A necessary preliminary approach to this problem is to localize the positions of amino acid sequence variation between different alleles of the α and β chains of Ia molecules, in order to determine whether they are clustered, or scattered throughout the entire polypeptide chain. The first approach to this question was to determine the nucleotide sequence of cDNA clones for A_α chains of the H-$2^{k,d,b,f,u,q}$ alleles. These results have been described in detail by Benoist *et al.* (1983b). The findings are given in summary form in Table 2.1(a) which presents the positions of allelic variations in the murine A_α immune response gene product from six different haplotypes. In the first domain, stretches of variant (allelic hypervariable) residues are seen at amino acids 10–15, 44–49, 53–59, 68–79. At most of these positions, several different amino acid residues occur. Isolated positions in which one variant or at most two variants are seen, occur at positions 28, 35, 66 and 83. In the second domain, there are only a few changes from the prototype sequence, in which one other amino acid is found at residues 133, 142, 147 and 175.

Table 2.1(a) also shows the allelic variability in three A_β polypeptides from the H-$2^{b,d,k}$ haplotypes determined by Choi *et al.* (1983). Table 2.1(b) presents the comparison of the E_α^k sequence determined in this laboratory (Benoist *et al.*, 1983a) with that of McNicholas *et al.* (1982) for the E_α^d allele. Table 2.1(b) also presents the comparison of the E_β^d sequence of Saito *et al.* (1983) with the E_β^k sequence of Mengle-Gaw & McDevitt (1983). From an examination of this table, several preliminary conclusions can be drawn, which may require modification when additional allelic sequence data become available.

First, the A_α, A_β and E_β polypeptide chains all exhibit an identical pattern of allelic variation. This allelic variation is localized to the first (external, amino-terminal and membrane-distal) domain. Within the first domain, allelic sequence variation tends to occur in 3-4 'allelic hypervariable' regions. [See footnote to Table 2.1(b) for a definition of 'allelic

Table 2.1. Regions of allelic hypervariability in murine I-A and I-E molecules*

(a) The I-A molecule

	A_{α_1} [6]†	A_{α_2} [6]
10–15	(3/6)‡	—
44–49	(3/6)§	—
53–59	(4/7)§	—
68–79	(5/9)	—
Total hypervariable residues	15	0
Isolated variants	4	4

	A_{β_1} [3]	A_{β_2} [3]
10–18	(5/9)¶	—
63–68	(4/6. 2 gaps)	—
85–90	(3/6)	—
Total hypervariable residues	12 + 2 gaps	0
Isolated variants	6	4

(b) The I-E molecule

	E_{α_1} [2]	E_{α_2} [2]
Hypervariable residues	0	0
Isolated variants	1	1

	E_{β_1} [2]	E_{β_2} [2]
1–13	(7/13)	—
24–35	(6/12)	—
68–75	(4/8)	—
Total hypervariable residues	17	0
Isolated variants	5	1

* A region of allelic hypervariability was arbitrarily defined as any stretch of six or more amino acid residues in which at least 50% of the positions exhibited allelic variation.

† This number indicates the number of alleles for which complete or nearly complete sequence information is available.

‡ This number gives the number of variant residues/total number of residues in a hypervariable stretch.

§ Combining these adjacent regions results in a single hypervariable stretch from residues 48–59 in which 5/12 residues vary.

¶ The first six residues are not yet sequenced (Choi *et al.*, 1983).

hypervariable' regions.] The spacing of these hypervariable regions, and their size, are roughly comparable to the hypervariable regions of immunoglobulin variable region sequences.

Second, A_α appears to be somewhat more variable than A_β. In contrast, E_β is clearly much more variable than E_α, which shows almost complete sequence conservation.

Thus, A_α, A_β and E_β can be characterized as having constant regions which consist of the second domain, the connecting peptide, and the transmembrane and cytoplasmic regions, and a variable first domain, within which there are 3-4 'allelic hypervariable' regions with a size and spacing similar to the hypervariable regions found in immunoglobulin V region sequences.

This finding naturally leads to the speculation that these allelic hypervariable regions are functionally important structures in regulating the immune response (McDevitt, 1981; Klein *et al.*, 1981). It is possible that they are associated with each other by the three-dimensional juxtaposition of allelic hypervariable regions by the folding of the first domain to form an 'active site'. This possibility is presented schematically in Fig. 2.3. This 'active site' may interact directly with foreign antigen on the surface of the antigen-presenting cell and on the B cell.

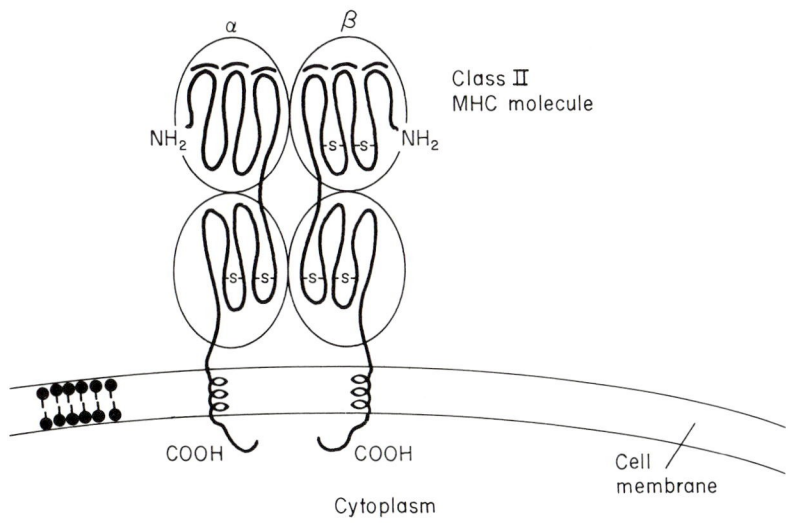

Fig. 2.3. Schematic diagram of the postulated arrangement of the α and β chain allelic hypervariable region (indicated by arcs), might be juxtaposed to form an I-A 'active site'.

These results leave many unanswered questions. How can a single I-A or I-E 'active site' regulate the response to many different antigens (McDevitt, 1981; Klein *et al.*, 1981)? While this might be due to a 'forced' interaction (in which only that part of the foreign antigen not in direct association with the 'active site' is 'seen' by the T cell receptor), such an interaction has yet to be demonstrated to occur on the surface of the antigen-presenting cell.

Second, and more closely related to the results presented here, is the question of the three-dimensional configuration of I-A and I-E molecules. This question, and the related question of the structure of the T cell receptor, are now the crucial issues in understanding how immune response genes work.

Acknowledgment

This work was supported by Grants AI 07757 and AI 18367 from the National Institutes of Health.

References

Altman, P. L. & Katz, D. D., eds (1979) *Adaptive Differentiation of Murine Lympocytes: Implications for Mechanisms of Cell–Cell Recognition and the Regulation of Immune Response*, Part 1. Federation of American Societies for Experimental Biology, Bethesda, Maryland.

Benacerraf, B. & Dorf, M. E. (1976) Genetic control of specific immune responses and immune suppressions by I-region genes. *Cold Spring Harbor Symp. quant. Biol.* **41**, 465.

Benoist, C. O., Mathis, D. J., Kanter, M. R., Williams, V. E. II, & McDevitt, H. O. (1983a) The murine Ia alpha chains, E alpha and A alpha, show a surprising degree of sequence homology. *Proc. natn. Acad. Sci. U.S.A.* **80**, 534.

Benoist, C. O., Mathis, D. J., Kanter, M. R., Williams, V. E. II, & McDevitt, H. O. (1983b) Regions of allelic hypervariability in the murine A alpha immune response gene. *Cell*, **34**, 169.

Choi, E., McIntyre, K., Germain, R. N. & Seidman, J. G. (1983) Murine I-A beta chain polymorphism: nucleotide sequences of three allelic I-A beta genes. *Science*, **211**, 283.

Das, H., Lawrence, S. & Weissman, S. M. (1983) Structure and nucleotide sequence of the heavy chain gene of HLA-DR. *Proc. natn. Acad. Sci. U.S.A.* **12**, 3543.

Duncan, W. R., Wakeland, E. K. & Klein, J. (1979) Histocompatibility 2 system in wild mice. *Immunogenetics*, **9**, 261.

Fuhrman, S. A., Deininger, P. L., La Porte, P., Friedman, T. & Guiduschek, P. (1981) Analysis of transcription of the human Alu family ubiquitous repeating element by eukargotic RNA polymerase III. *Nucleic Acids Res.* **9**, 995.

Jones, P., Murphy, D. & McDevitt, H. O. (1981) Variable synthesis and expression of Eπ and Ae (Eeβ) Ia polypeptide chains in mice of different H-2 haplotype. *Immunogenetics*, **12**, 321.

Klein, J., Juretic, A., Bazevanis, C. N. & Nagy, Z. A. (1981) The traditional and a new version of the mouse H-2 complex. *Nature (Lond.)*, **291**, 455.

Klein, J., Merryman, C. F., Maurer, P. H., Hauptfeld, M. & Gerdner, M. B. (1976) Histocompatibility-2 system of wild mice. IV. Ia and Ir typing of two wild mouse populations. *Cold Spring Harbor Symp. quant. Biol.* **41**, 457.

McDevitt, H. O. (1981) The role of H-2 I region gene in regulation of the immune response. *J. Immunogenet.* **8**, 287.

McNicholas, J., Steinmetz, M., Hu Kappi, J., Jones, P. & Hood, L. (1982) DNA sequence of the gene encoding the E$_\alpha$ Ia polypeptide of the BALB/c mouse. *Science*, **218**, 1229.

Mathis, D. J., Benoist, C., Williams, V. E. II, Kanter, M. R. & McDevitt, H. O. (1983a) Several mechanisms can account for defective E alpha gene expression in different mouse haplotypes. *Proc. natn. Acad. Sci. U.S.A.* **80**, 273.

Mathis, D. J., Benoist, C. O., Williams, V. E. II, Kanter, M. R. & McDevitt, H. O. (1983b) The murine E alpha immune response gene. *Cell*, **32**, 745.

Maxman, A. & Gilbert, W. (1980) Sequencing end-labeled DNA with base specific chemical cleavages. *Methods Enzymol.* **65**, 499.

Mengle-Gaw, L. & McDevitt, H. O. (1983) Isolation and characterisation of C DNA clone for the murine I-E polypeptide chain. *Proc. natn. Acad. Sci. U.S.A.* **80**, 7621.

Nagy, Z., Baxevanis, C., Ishii, N. & Klein, J. (1981) Ia antigens as restriction molecules in Ir gene controlled T cell proliferation. *Immunol. Rev.* **60**, 59.

Rosenthal, A. (1978) Determinant selection and macrophage function in genetic control of the immune response. *Immunol. Rev.* **40**, 136.

Saito, H., Maki, R. A., Clayton, L. K. & Tonegawa, S. (1983) Complete primary structures of the E beta chain and gene of the mouse major histocompatibility complex. *Proc. natn. Acad. Sci. U.S.A.* (in press).

Sanger, F., Coulson, A. R., Barrell, B. G., Smith, A. J. H. & Roe, B. A. (1980) Cloning in single-stranded bacteriophage as an aid to rapid DNA sequencing. *J. molec. Biol.* **143**, 161.

Schwartz, R. H., David, C. S., Sachs, D. H. & Paul, W. E. (1976) T lymphocyte-enriched murine peritoneal exudate cells. III. Inhibition of antigen induced T lymphocyte proliferation with anti-Ia antisera. *J. Immunol.* **117**, 531.

Solinger, A. M., Ultee, M. E., Margoliash, E. & Schwartz, R. H. (1979) Lymphocyte response to cytochrome. *J. exp. Med.* **150**, 830.

Chapter 3
The significance of MHC restriction

B. Benacerraf & K. L. Rock

Department of Pathology, Harvard Medical School, 25 Shattuck Street,
Boston, Massachusetts 02130, U.S.A.

Summary. The significance of MHC restriction of specific T lymphocytes was investigated in relation to: (i) the origin of alloreactivity; (ii) the presentation of antigen by Ia-bearing accessory cells. Alloreactivity and the commitment of large fractions of T cells to reactivity with allo-MHC antigens will be shown to be the unavoidable consequence of the commitment of T cells to recognize foreign antigens together with autologous MHC molecules. Evidence will also be presented of the interaction of Ia molecules and foreign antigens at the surface of accessory cells before specific interactions of the complex with the T cells.

Introduction

We owe to Peter Gorer and to George Snell (Gorer, Lyman & Snell, 1948) the discovery that the rejection of tissue transplants between two incompatible individuals of the same species is the result of a specific immunological reaction directed against highly polymorphic antigens expressed on the surface of cells. They called the membrane components, against which anti-graft immunity is directed, histocompatibility antigens. Furthermore Gorer and Snell (Gorer *et al.*, 1948) made the critical discovery that the strongest histocompatibility antigens, in the mouse, are coded for by a group of closely linked loci which they named H-2, the murine major histocompatibility complex (MHC).

The MHC has since presented a considerable challenge, as it is evident that the rejection of allografts does not have survival value and therefore that this complex system did not evolve for this trivial purpose. The development of this complex system of genes must have some other very important evolutionary significance and function. The answer to this question was provided by experiments in a completely different field from transplantation immunology, resulting in the discovery of immune response (Ir) genes (Levine, Ojeda & Benacerraf, 1963) and the demonstration that Ir genes code for transplantation antigens of the major histocompatibility complex (McDevitt & Chinitz, 1969). The finding that

MHC molecules are selectively concerned with the specific activation of T lymphocytes (Benacerraf & McDevitt, 1972) stimulated studies of the specificity of T lymphocytes and of their regulatory interactions with other cells of the immune system, where MHC antigens play a critical role.

The following points have been clearly established.

1 MHC antigens are concerned with our ability to distinguish self from non-self.

2 T lymphocytes develop receptors for self MHC antigens during differentiation; however, only mature T cells, with specific receptors of low affinity against self MHC, are allowed to migrate from the thymus (Bevan, 1977).

3 T cells react to conventional foreign antigens only when presented on cell surfaces in conjunction with autologous MHC antigens (Shevach & Rosenthal, 1973; Zinkernagel & Doherty, 1975).

4 MHC molecules, therefore, govern the necessary cell interactions concerned with antigen-induced stimulation between the various cells of the immune system, T cells, B cells (Katz, Hamaoka & Benacerraf, 1973) and macrophages (Shevach & Rosenthal, 1973).

5 The extensive polymorphism of MHC antigens has as its consequence that individuals differ in their ability to respond specifically to selected antigens, which is the basis of Ir gene phenomenology (Benacerraf & McDevitt, 1972).

The commitment of T lymphocytes to recognizing foreign antigens on the surface of cells only when presented in the context of MHC molecules, raised many important questions currently investigated by numerous immunologists. My laboratory has been more particularly concerned, in the last few years, with three aspects of the significance of MHC restriction: (i) the generation, in the thymus, of T lymphocyte populations with receptors for autologous MHC antigens; (ii) the origin of alloreactivity; and (iii) the basis for the specificity of Ir gene function.

Development of thymocytes reactive with autologous MHC antigens

The thymus is an organ necessary for the maturation of functional T lymphocytes (Miller & Osoba, 1964). In this organ, striking T cell proliferation and cell death are observed. It has been generally assumed that these phenomena are in some way responsible for the generation and selection of a mature T cell population (Stutman, 1978), comprising cells with distinct receptors, yet they are all specifically able to bind foreign antigens in the context of self MHC molecules. Our experiments were based on the premise that this process must take place in two stages: (i) T cells with receptors for self MHC antigens are stimulated in the thymus to differentiate and proliferate (Zinkernagel, 1978); (ii) only those T cells which bear low affinity receptors for self MHC antigens can mature and leave the thymus as functional T cells.

We further postulated that the first process of selection and proliferation of thymocytes reactive with autologous MHC antigens should proceed by the same mechanism which triggers mature peripheral T cells, that is, as a consequence of specific interaction with Ia-bearing autologous accessory cells, resulting in the stimulation of interleukin-1 (IL-1) secretion by these cells (Rock & Benacerraf, submitted). We considered that the classical IL-1 assay, based on the proliferation of thymocytes to IL-1, is a reflection of this process. We therefore investigated whether the proliferative response of thymocytes to IL-1 is absolutely dependent on the presence of Ia-bearing accessory cells. As shown in Table 3.1, the response of thymocytes to IL-1 is significantly inhibited if the responding population is treated with an appropriately specific monoclonal anti-Ia antibody and complement, or passed through nylon wool to eliminate Ia-bearing accessory cells. Moreover, Ia-bearing accessory cells, with equivalent capacity to promote the response of thymocytes to IL-1, exist equally in the low density fraction of the spleen and of the thymus (Rock & Benacerraf, submitted).

Table 3.1. The response of thymocytes to IL-1 requires Ia-bearing accessory cells

Thymocyte* treatment	X-irradiated[†] nylon wool-adherent	IL-1[‡]	c.p.m.
None	−	−	552
None	−	+	25,413
Anti-Ia + C§	−	−	182
Anti-Ia + C	−	+	5823
Anti-Ia + C	+	−	266
Anti-Ia + C	+	+	21,272

* 1.5×10^6 BALB/c thymocytes.
† 2×10^5 nylon wool adherent + 1660 rads.
‡ 1:8 supernatant dilution.
§ Nylon wool-passed and anti-Ia antibody and complement (C)-treated.

These findings led us to explore: (i) whether IL-1 was produced in supernatants of cultures of thymocytes with thymic or splenic accessory cells, and (ii) whether thymocytes were induced to proliferate in these cultures in the absence of added IL-1. The results of these experiments (data not shown) were very conclusive. IL-1 activity was readily demonstrable in supernatants of cultures of thymocytes with accessory cells. Furthermore, thymocyte proliferation was observed to coincide in time with the intrinsic production of IL-1 in the culture. Both the production of IL-1 and the proliferative response of thymocytes could be inhibited by the deletion of Ia-bearing accessory cells (using anti-Ia antibody and complement) or by the addition of appropriately specific monoclonal anti-Ia antibody to the cultures. A comparison of the proliferative responses of medullary and cortical thymocytes revealed a stronger response by the more mature medullary thymocytes (Rock & Benacerraf, 1984b). We concluded from these experiments that the proliferation, which is normally observed in the thymus, reflects the stimulation and expansion of clones specific for self class II MHC molecules. These clones react with Ia molecules on thymic accessory cells and stimulate them to secrete IL-1, which in turn acts as the second requisite signal for thymocyte proliferation.

As a consequence of these findings, the prediction can be made that thymocytes, in contrast to peripheral T cells, comprise a relatively high fraction of cells reactive with autologous class II MHC antigens, in the absence of foreign antigens. Moreover, if allowed to escape as functional mature T cells to the secondary lymphoid organs, these cells could cause considerable damage, and probably initiate autologous graft-versus-host disease. There must therefore be a second very important mechanism for the selective deletion after the initial expansion of those T cells with high affinity for autologous MHC antigens. There is, however, no information at present on the precise nature of this critical process in the maturation of T cells except for a recent report from Glazier *et al.* (1983). These authors made the intriguing observation that if they treated heavily irradiated rats with cyclosporin, previous to reconstitution with syngeneic bone marrow cells, these animals, in contrast to untreated animals that reconstituted normally, developed severe graft-versus-host disease, in spite of having received only syngeneic or autologous bone marrow cells. It would appear, therefore, that the process whereby the maturing high affinity thymocytes, reactive with autologous MHC antigens, are normally deleted or sequestred is in some way sensitive to cyclosporin in the rat.

The origin of alloreactivity

The origin of alloreactivity has always been a considerable puzzle to immunologists as soon as it was realized that a relatively large fraction of mature T cells are reactive with alloantigens of the MHC (Wilson, Blyth & Nowell, 1968). Such a large fraction of alloreactive T lymphocytes was not easily compatible with the reactivity of T cells with the numerous T-dependent foreign antigens for which they are specific, unless the same T cell populations are responsible for both reactivities (Jerne, 1971). The discovery that T cells only react to foreign antigens in the context of autologous MHC antigens permitted this problem to be addressed at the clonal level. We postulated that, after the deletion of the T cells reactive with autologous MHC antigens with high affinity (discussed in the previous section), the remaining T cells with low affinity for self MHC antigens should display high affinity for slight variants of self MHC

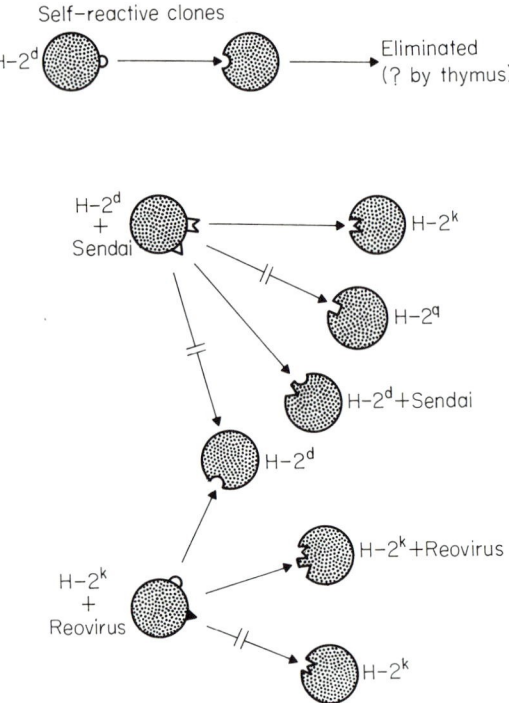

Fig. 3.1. Graphic representation illustrating that a cytolytic T cell clone, specific for Sendai virus, is capable of killing syngeneic virally infected target cells or uninfected allogeneic target cells of the appropriate haplotype.

antigens expressed in the same species. These clones should in fact be heteroclitic with respect to alloMHC antigens. Moreover, the same clone should be reactive with selfMHC + x and with a particular alloMHC antigen. A different clone selected with reactivity to selfMHC + y should express reactivity for a different alloMHC antigen (Lemonnier *et al.*, 1977).

According to this hypothesis, alloreactivity and the apparent commitment of large fraction of T cells to reactivity with alloMHC antigens is the unavoidable result of the commitment of T cells to recognize foreign antigens together with autologous MHC antigens, and the concomitant deletion of those clones with high affinity for self MHC antigens.

This hypothesis has been verified in every one of its predictions. Initially with my colleagues Finberg, Burakoff and Cantor (Finberg *et al.*, 1978), we demonstrated that Sendai-immunized BALB/c mice developed cytolytic T cells capable of killing Sendai-infected H-2^d target cells and also non-infected allogeneic target cells. Cold target competition experiments revealed that different T cell clones, each specific for Sendai and H-2^d, were lytic for different uninfected allogeneic targets. This experiment is graphically illustrated in Fig. 3.1. Our experiments were confirmed and extended with both class I and class II MHC-restricted, antigen-specific, T cell clones, formally demonstrating that both specificities, self + x and alloreactivity, are the property of a single specific T cell.

Basis for specificity of MHC restriction of T cells

The specificity of T cells for self MHC antigens in conjunction with foreign antigens determines restrictions in the ability of T cells to react with these foreign molecules, so that animals with certain MHC haplotypes are responders and others with other MHC haplotypes are non-responders to the same antigen (Benacerraf & McDevitt, 1972). This behaviour, which is the basis of Ir gene phenomenology, has been noted for both class I and class II MHC antigens, although it has been most extensively studied for class I Ia antigens, the original Ir gene products.

Two types of explanation have been proposed to account for the manner in which MHC molecules affect the specific pattern of immune reactivity of T lymphocytes.

(i) Rosenthal, Barcinski & Blake (1977) and Benacerraf (1978) postulated that the interaction of Ia molecules with foreign antigens on the surface of antigen-presenting cells posed certain restrictions on the preferential orientation of these molecules and restricted their ability to bind to T cell specific receptors, thus introducing the concept of determinant selection of foreign antigens, as a consequence of Ia molecule–antigen interactions. The major criticism directed against this hypothesis is the lack of heterogeneity in Ia molecules in any given individual. Two classes of Ia molecules exist, and in any individual heterozygous at these loci there can be at most eight molecules. This number of eight distinct Ia molecules may appear to be too small to account for the extent of Ir gene-specific restrictions observed.

(ii) The other hypothesis, proposed by von Boehmer, Hass & Jerne (1978) and modified by Schwartz (1978), postulates that the Ir gene defects are the result of clonal deletion at the level of the T cell. During differentiation, when T cells are rendered tolerant to self antigen in relation to autologous MHC antigens, certain foreign antigens plus self MHC molecules mimic some autologous molecule in the context of the same self MHC molecules. This results in the deletion of the corresponding T cell clones and in the inability to respond to the relevant foreign antigens for animals with these MHC haplotypes. This hypothesis is indeed very attractive but difficult to prove. Nevertheless, it must be emphasized that the two mechanisms proposed are not mutually exclusive and may very well both be correct.

Several lines of experimentation have supported the model of Ia molecule–antigen interaction at the level of the antigen-presenting cell proposed by Rosenthal et al. (1977) and ourselves (1978). Perhaps the most persuasive evidence stems from the analysis of determinant selection phenomena. Experiments by Herber-Katz et al. (1982) using T cell hybridomas have shown that the Ia molecules on the antigen-presenting cells are, in selected cases, responsible for the response or non-response of a T cell cloned line to a particular epitope on an Ir gene-controlled antigen.

Our laboratory has also addressed the issue of Ia molecule–antigen interaction by documenting the existence of antigen competition at the antigen-presenting cell level between related antigens under Ir gene control. Indeed the specific association model makes a unique prediction. If there are a limited number of binding sites on Ia molecules, then more than one antigen will utilize the same site, resulting in antigen competition. The first demonstration that this prediction is correct was contributed by Werdelin (1982). Using a guinea-pig T cell proliferation assay and uncloned T cell populations, he showed competition, localized to the antigen-presenting cell between GL and DNP-PLL, two antigens with the same responder status in strain-2 guinea-pigs.

We felt that the analysis of specific antigenic competition would be more informative if we used T cell hybridomas and clonal accessory cells (APC), thereby avoiding the potential complications inherent in the heterogeneity of uncloned T cell populations with multiple specificities (Rock & Benacerraf, 1983a). We selected several H-2^d-restricted T cell hybridomas specific for the co-polymer of L-glutamic acid, L-alanine and L-tyrosine (GAT), and investigated the effect of the structurally related co-polymers GT and GA on the activation of these hybridomas. Neither of these structurally related co-polymers can activate these GAT-specific hybridomas. However, we made the striking observation that inclusion of the non-responder co-polymer GT in cultures of RF9.140 (a representative cloned line) with GAT and syngeneic APC markedly inhibited activation of the T cell hybridomas (Rock & Benacerraf, 1983a). To define further the specificity of inhibition, we tested the effect of addition of unrelated co-polymers and did not detect any inhibition. Furthermore, GT was shown to have no effect on the activation of T cell clone of other specificities.

We then undertook to define the site of competition between the antigens GT and GAT. Experiments were performed where either the accessory cells or the T cell hybridomas were preincubated with GT and then tested for functional activity. We noted that, if BALB/c accessory cells are pulsed with GAT for 18 hr and subsequently washed to remove free antigen, they will function to activate RF9.140. However, if GT is present during the preincubation period, there is marked interference with effective antigen pulsing. We have repeated this experiment using the A-20 antigen-presenting B cell line as APC, and we have shown that GT interferes with the ability of this cell to present GAT to the T cell hybridoma. The reciprocal experiment, where the T cell hybridoma is preincubated with GT previous to interaction with GAT-pulsed antigen-presenting cells (APC), showed no inhibition, indicating that the mechanism of inhibition is not the result of interaction of free antigen with the T cell receptor. Taken together, these results illustrate a highly specific inhibition between two structurally related antigens for appropriate presentation by an antigen-presenting cell. The results further suggest that inhibition occurs after antigen uptake and processing.

We next investigated the involvement of MHC gene products in this competition. We tested the effect of GT upon responses of GAT-specific hybrids restricted to I-A^d versus I-A^b. We observed that GT inhibits the I-A^d-restricted hybrids, but not the I-A^b-restricted hybrids. This selective inhibition is also observed if F$_1$(d × b) APCs are used, demonstrating that

Table 3.2. Inhibition by GT of the response to GAT of a representative BALB/c × BW5147 GAT-specific T cell hybrid

| Hybrid* | 18 hr pulse of A-20 APC† | | | |
	25 g/ml GAT	200 g/ml OVA	100 g/ml GT	c.p.m.
RF9.140	−	−	−	258
	+	+	−	21,429
	+	+	+	1622
DO11.10	−	−	−	218
	+	+	−	2145
	+	+	+	5380

* RF9.140 is a BALB/c anti-I-A^d + GAT hybrid. DO11.10 is a BALB/c anti-I-A^d + OVA hybrid (kindly provided by Drs J. Kappler and P. Marrack).

† A-20 is a BALB/c I-A + B lymphoblastoid line.

the particular allele of the I-A restriction element determines in some manner the susceptibility to GT competition at the level of the APC. These data are consistent with the specific association model we proposed, where different Ia molecules have different binding sites for a given antigen, such as GAT.

We then addressed the issue of antigen Ia interaction by a different approach (Rock & Benacerraf, 1983b). If there is indeed specific association of antigen with Ia molecules, then a specific portion of an Ia molecule will be complexed and hence blocked or modified by antigen. An alloreactive T cell, selected with specificity for the relevant interaction site on the Ia molecule, might be able to detect such an association. Such alloreactive T cells should be inhibitable in their specific interaction with Ia, by the relevant nominal antigen. We developed, accordingly, a series of alloreactive I-A^d-specific T cell hybridomas and analysed the effect of GAT on the activation of these hybrids. We were able to identify one of these anti-I-A^d hybridomas (RF19.24) which was inhibited by GAT. This inhibition was specific, as several other identically derived I-A^d hybrids, were not inhibited by GAT. Both GAT and GT were equally inhibitory of the activation of RF19.24 by I-A^d, while GA and other antigens were without effect. We interpreted these results as indicating that, as an APC interacts with GAT or GT, it may lose the ability to present a particular I-A allodeterminant to the appropriately specific T cell clone, while it gains the capacity to present GAT to other T cell clones. Thus, RF19.24 may recognize an I-A epitope involved in or in proximity to a GAT association site or alternatively, the interaction of I-A^d with GAT results in a change of configuration which deletes the epitope recognized by RF19.24. Both explanations imply that there has been a specific interaction between Ia and GAT on the antigen-presenting cell.

These experiments, taken together with our studies of antigenic competition, support therefore the concept we proposed of specific antigen–Ia association. We feel that the specific association we have documented, with selected antigens, constitutes a general mechanism utilized in the presentation of antigens to T cells, and explains in a large measure the contribution of MHC molecules to the phenomena of Ir gene specificity. These data, however, are not incompatible with the possibility that in selected cases MHC-controlled non-responsiveness may result from deletion in the T cell repertoire, as suggested recently by Ishii, Nagy & Klein (1982). It is most reasonable to conclude, therefore, that both mechanisms contribute to the manner in which MHC restrictions control the specificity of T cells for foreign antigen.

Acknowledgment

This work was supported by Grants AI-14732 and 1 RO1-AI-CA-20248-01, from the National Institute of Allergy and Infectious Diseases, National Institutes of Health.

References

Benacerraf, B. (1978) A hypothesis to relate the specificity of T-lymphocytes and the reactivity of I region specific IR genes in macrophages and B lymphocytes. *J. Immunol.* **120**, 1809.

Benacerraf, B. & McDevitt, H. O. (1972) The histocompatibility linked immune response genes. *Science*, **175**, 273.

Bevan, M. (1977) In a radiation chimera, host H-2 antigens determine immune responsiveness of donor cytotoxic cells. *Nature (Lond.)*, **269**, 417.

Finberg, R., Burakoff, S. J., Cantor, H. & Benacerraf, B. (1978) The biological significance of alloreactivity. T cells stimulated by Sendai virus coated syngeneic cells specifically lyse allogeneic targets cells. *Proc. natn Acad. Sci. U.S.A.* **75**, 5145.

Glazier, A., Tutschka, P. J., Farmer, E. R. & Santos, G. W. (1983) Graft-versus-host disease in cyclosporin A treated rats after syngeneic and autologous bone marrow reconstitution. *J. exp. Med.* **158**, 1.

Gorer, P. A., Lyman, S. & Snell, G. D. (1948) Studies on the genetic and antigenic basis of tumour transplantation. Linkage between a histocompatibility gene and 'fused' in mice. *Proc. R. Soc. (Biol.)*, **135**, 499.

Heber-Katz, E., Schwartz, R. H., Matis, L. A., Hannum, C., Fairwell, T., Apella, E. & Hansburg, D. (1982) Contribution of antigen-presenting cell major histocompatibility complex gene products to the specificity of antigen-induced T cell activation. *J. exp. Med.* **155**, 1086.

Ishii, N., Nagy, L. A. & Klein, J. (1982) Restriction molecules involved in the interaction of T cells with allogeneic antigen-presenting cells. *J. exp. Med.* **156**, 622.

Jerne, N. K. (1971). The somatic generation of immune recognition. *Eur. J. Immunol.* **1**, 1.

Katz, D. H., Hamaoka, T., & Benacerraf, B. (1973) Cell interaction between histocompatible T and B lymphocytes. II. Failure of cooperative interactions between T and B lymphocytes from allogeneic donor strains in humoral response to hapten-protein conjugates. *J. exp. Med.* **137**, 1405.

Lemonnier, F., Burakoff, S., Germain, R. & Benacerraf, B. (1977) Cytolytic T lymphocytes specific for allogeneic stimulator cells cross-react with chemically modified syngeneic cells. *Proc. natn. Acad. Sci. U.S.A.* **74**, 1229.

Levine, B. B., Ojeda, A., & Benacerraf, B. (1963). Studies on artificial antigens. The genetic control of the immune response to hapten poly-L-lysine conjugates in guinea-pigs. *J. exp. Med.* **118**, 953.

McDevitt, H. O. & Chinitz, A. (1969) Genetic control of antibody response: relationship between immune response and histocompatibility (H-2) type. *Science*, **163**, 1207.

Miller, J. F. A. P. & Osoba, D. (1964) Current concepts of the immunological function of the thymus. *Phys. Rev.* **47**, 437.

Rock, K. L. & Benacerraf, B. (1983a) Inhibition of antigen specific T lymphocyte activation by structurally related Ir gene controlled polymers: evidence of specific competition for accessory cell antigen presentation. *J. exp. Med.* **157**, 1618.

Rock, K. L. & Benacerraf, B. (1983b) MHC restricted T cell activation: analysis with T cell hybridomas. *Immunol. Rev.* (in press).

Rock, K. L. & Benacerraf, B. (1984a) The role of Ia molecules in the activation of T lymphocytes. IV. The basis of the thymocyte IL-1 response and its possible role in the generation of the T cell repertoire. *J. Immunol.* (submitted).

Rock, K. L. & Benacerraf, B. (1984b) Thymic T cells are driven to expand upon interaction with self-class II MHC gene products on accessory cells. *Proc. natn Acad. Sci. U.S.A.* (in press).

Rosenthal, A. S., Barcinski, A. M. & Blake, T. J. (1977) Determinant selection is a macrophage dependent immune response gene function. *Nature (Lond.)*, **267**, 156.

Schwartz, R. H. (1978) A clonal deletion model for Ir gene control of the immune response. *Scand. J. Immunol.* **7**, 3.

Shevach, E. M. & Rosenthal, A. S. (1973) Function of macrophages in antigen recognition by guinea pig lymphocytes. II. Role of macrophages in the regulation of genetic control of the immune response. *J. exp. Med.* **138**, 1213.

Stutman, O. (1978) Intrathymic and extrathymic T cell maturation. *Immunol. Rev.* **42**, 138.

von Boehmer, H., Haas, W. & Jerne, N. K. (1978) Major histocompatibility complex-linked immune responsiveness is acquired by lymphocytes of low responder mice differentiating in thymus of high responder mice. *Proc. natn. Acad. Sci. U.S.A.* **75**, 2439.

Werdelin, O. (1982) Chemically related antigens compete for presentation by accessory cells to T cell. *J. Immunol.* **129**, 1883.

Wilson, D. B., Blyth, J. L. & Nowell, P. C. (1968) Quantitative studies of the mixed lymphocyte interaction in rats. III. Kinetics of the response. *J. exp. Med.* **128**, 1157.

Zinkernagel, R. M. (1978) Thymus and lymphohemopoietic cells: their role in the T cell maturation in selection of T cells' H-2 restriction specificity and in H-2 linked Ir gene control. *Immunol. Rev.* **42**, 224.

Zinkernagel, R. M. & Doherty, P. C. (1975) H-2 histocompatibility requirement for T cell mediated lysis of target cells infected with choriomeningitis virus. Different cytotoxic cell specificities are associated with structures coded for in H-2K or H-2D. *J. exp. Med.* **141**, 1427.

Chapter 4
Concepts of immunological enhancement

J. R. Batchelor

Department of Immunology, Royal Postgraduate Medical School,
Hammersmith Hospital, Du Cane Road, London W12 0HS

Summary. Indefinitely prolonged survival of orthotopic kidney allografts can be induced in many rat strains by active or passive immunological enhancement regimens. The prolonged survival can occur even when donor and recipient strains differ at the major histocompatibility system loci, and in many donor/recipient combinations, the enhanced graft survival does not require the use of non-specific immunosuppressive measures.

Experiments are described which show that enhanced kidney grafts lose a population of highly immunogenic passenger cells, which include dendritic cells. This is one major factor leading to the extended graft survival. A second factor is the induction of suppressor T cells; the activity of these may not be discerned unless the assay system consists of testing for suppression of rejection of a kidney allograft that has been depleted of highly immunogenic passenger cells.

Introduction

This article reviews experimental work on which the author's present concepts of immunological enhancement are based. To a large extent the work described is that from the author's own laboratory, and is not a comprehensive review of the whole field of enhancement. As the occasion is a symposium dedicated to Peter Gorer, a personal account seemed appropriate.

For those unfamiliar with the phenomenon of immunological enhancement, it may be useful to start by defining it. In his superb review, Kaliss (1958) stated that it is the establishment and progressive growth of a tumour graft as a consequence of the tumour's contact with specific antiserum in the host. The presence of antiserum may result from passive or active immunization. However, this definition has become unsatisfactory, as will become evident later.

Early observations on enhancement in the first half of this century

28

were based on experimental systems involving the use of transplantable tumours. A consequence was that the phenomenon became identified with the growth of tumours. Such thinking was of course flabby logic, as had been pointed out by Peter Gorer (1961).

Thus, the question of whether normal tissue grafts could also manifest immunological enhancement was not raised until during the '50s, and because enhancement of normal tissues such as skin or ovarian grafts was frequently either undramatic or not demonstrable, the potential importance of this issue was not widely appreciated.

A number of developments changed attitudes. The first was the introduction of a practical immunosuppressive therapy and the start of clinical renal transplant programmes. Secondly, there was the pioneering work by Lee (1967) on microvascular surgery for experimental animal models. Lastly, inbred rat strains became more widely available. Thus the possibility of developing vascularized organ allograft models in genetically defined animal strains coincided with an appreciation of its need. Whether immunological enhancement was an effective means of preventing the rejection of normal tissue could then be asked of an orthotopic kidney allograft. As reported some years ago, French & Batchelor (1969) demonstrated the indefinite survival of $(AS \times AUG)F_1$ kidneys after transplantation into AS recipients passively immunized with AS anti-August antiserum (so called passive enhancement). Control animals, not injected with the antiserum, always rejected the RT1 incompatible grafts and died with 12 days.

The natural history of rat kidney graft enhancement

Immunological status of the recipient

A number of questions suggested themselves, foremost of which was the immunological status of the rats with the long-surviving, enhanced kidneys. It appeared that the rats passed through an inductive phase of enhancement during the first 2–3 weeks after transplantation, followed by a maintenance phase which persisted (Batchelor & Welsh, 1976; Batchelor, Welsh & Burgos, 1977b). During the inductive phase, the IgM alloantibody response seen in controls was entirely absent, a variable reduction in the IgG alloantibody response occurred, and there was a delay in the generation of the cytotoxic T cell response. Depending on a number of factors, which included the amount of enhancing antiserum given, the abnormal host response failed to cause graft destruction, although clinical, biochemical, and histological evidence of some graft damage during this period was usual.

At approximately 14–21 days after transplantation, the abortive rejection response resolves, and the rats enter the maintenance phase in which they become cumulatively less responsive to AUG strain alloantigens. Immunological memory, IgG antibody responses, and generation of cytotoxic T cells reactive with donor targets are markedly inhibited.

Interestingly, lymphocytes harvested from rats with long-surviving grafts can mount local GvH responses (French, Batchelor & Watts, 1971) or proliferative reactions *in vitro* (Batchelor *et al.*, 1977b) when confronted with donor alloantigens. Furthermore, if spleen or lymph node cells from AS rats immunized against AUG strain tissues are transferred to AS rats carrying long-surviving, enhanced (AS × AUG)F$_1$ kidney grafts, the transfer does not give rise to any signs of graft rejection, even though more than 30×10^8 cells were injected (Bowen *et al.*, 1974). Even if the hyperimmune AS rats were parabiosed for 9 days with syngeneic partners carrying long-surviving, enhanced kidneys, rejection of the grafts did not result. It was therefore concluded that an undefined 'suppressor' mechanism had developed in the long-term survivors which actively frustrated the specific rejection response.

At this point, attempts were made to detect suppressor cells in the long-term surviving rats. The obvious experiment was to transfer spleen cells from the rats with enhanced kidneys to immunologically naive syngeneic recipients which then were challenged with kidney allografts of the same genotype as the immunologically enhanced kidney. The author found that no suppressive effect was demonstrable with this model (unreported experiments), and Fabre & Morris (1972) reached the same conclusion in a different donor/recipient combination. Another system for looking for suppressor cell activity has been devised by Brent and his co-workers (Kilshaw & Brent, 1977); it consisted of the transfer of putative suppressor cells to a naive syngeneic host, immunosuppressed with anti-lymphocyte serum (ALS), and then challenging the recipient with a skin graft of the appropriate strain. Control immunosuppressed hosts recover immunological competence and reject the skin allografts at 20–40 days. However, following transfer of active suppressor cells, the return of immunologic competence is delayed and the skin allografts continue to survive, in some cases indefinitely. But even with this approach, we were unable to demonstrate the presence of suppressor cells in the spleens of AS rats carrying long-surviving, enhanced (AS × AUG)F$_1$ kidneys (Batchelor, Brent & Kilshaw, 1977a).

Summarizing the position at that time, we were led to conclude that a suppressor mechanism was responsible, at least in part, for the prolonged survival of the enhanced kidneys during the maintenance phase, but we had failed to unravel the details of the suppressor mechanism.

Immunogenicity of the enhanced kidney allograft

Until then, attention had been focused almost exclusively on the immunological status of the rat with the enhanced kidney. However, there was also the long-surviving graft to consider; was its immunogenicity modified by its residence in the recipient? Our earlier studies had shown that long-surviving grafts still expressed the original donor MHC antigens (Fine *et al.*, 1973), and more recent studies by Hart, Winnearls & Fabre (1980) demonstrated that the expression included both class I and II antigens. Nevertheless it seemed possible that despite the continued presence of alloantigens, graft immunogenicity may have been altered. Hints of this possibility had been given by model experiments in which allogeneic platelets, red cells, lymphocyte membranes and liposomes containing MHC antigens failed to induce strong, primary alloimmunity (Welsh, Burgos & Batchelor, 1977; Batchelor, Welsh & Burgos, 1978). It was therefore clear that the mere presence of MHC antigens of either class I or II was not enough to act as a strong primary alloimmunogen. Other factors must also be involved.

The direct way to test the immunogenicity of a long-surviving, enhanced kidney was to retransplant the graft into a second but naive recipient, syngeneic with the first. As previously reported (Batchelor *et al.*, 1979), a long-surviving, enhanced $(AS \times AUG)F_1$ kidney retransplanted from the first AS recipient into an otherwise untreated second AS rat survives for prolonged periods, and does not induce the normal T cell-dependent immune responses seen after grafting normal $(AS \times AUG)F_1$ kidneys. Indeed, when tested approximately 2 months after the retransplantation operation, the second recipient displays an identical non-responsiveness to that seen in the first.

The most probable explanation of the failure of the enhanced grafts to be rejected was thought to be because they had lost a subpopulation of highly immunogenic allogeneic passenger cells. Without the passenger cells, acute rejection was not induced in this donor/recipient combination. It was presumed that the original passenger cells of F_1 origin were replaced by AS passengers in the first recipient. Naturally the latter would not be incompatible when the F_1 kidney was retransplanted into the second AS recipient.

To test this hypothesis, we performed an experiment designed to prevent the passenger cell population being permanently replaced by AS cells in the first recipient (Lechler & Batchelor, 1982b). In brief, AS rats with enhanced F_1 grafts were made into chimeras by X-irradiation and injection of $(AS \times AUG)F_1$ bone marrow. Since any passenger cells in the graft are likely to be ultimately derived from bone marrow stem cells, this procedure should repopulate the graft with F_1 passengers and restore its immunogenicity to normal levels. Retransplantation into a second AS recipient should in that case be followed by a normal, acute rejection. The results of the experiment demonstrated that this indeed occurred, confirming that the immunogenicity of the graft depended chiefly on the genotype of its passenger cell population.

Identification of the subpopulation responsible for strong immuno-genicity was the next obvious task. The experimental design used was to retransplant an F_1 kidney into a second AS recipient as previously described, but at completion of the operation to inject purified subpopu-lations of F_1 cells thought to be part of the passenger cell population (Lechler & Batchelor, 1982a). It was found that acute rejection of the retransplanted F_1 kidney followed injection of small numbers of F_1 dendritic cells derived from afferent lymph by the method of Mason, Pugh & Webb (1981). Whereas $1-5 \times 10^4$ dendritic cells were able to trigger an acute rejection response, neither 5×10^6 F_1 T nor the same number of B lymphocytes were able to do so, indicating at least a 100-fold difference in immunogenicity. The immunogenicity of macrophage re-mained unresolved because of the heterogeneity of the populations we were able to prepare.

These results led to the following hypothesis. Primary alloimmuniza-tion can occur by two routes if the incompatibility involves the MHC. By route 1, viable allogeneic dendritic cells within a graft can bypass the need for further antigen processing because they are able to activate directly the recipient's T_H lymphocytes. Dendritic cells are postulated as being the only cells which can do this, a postulate strongly supported by the studies *in vitro* of Steinmann & Nussenzweig (1980) and Mason *et al.* (1981). Immunization can also proceed by route 2; here alloantigens of the graft are processed and presented by the recipient's own accessory cells, and events do not in principle differ from the handling and presentation of minor H system incompatibilities or conventional protein antigens.

For reasons which have been discussed in detail elsewhere (Lechler &

Batchelor, 1982a), route 1 is likely to be a highly efficient activation system, whereas route 2, although showing considerable variation, is much less efficient. According to our hypothesis, the crucial distinction between MHC-incompatible grafts and all other types of antigen is that the former, by virtue of their content of viable MHC-incompatible dendritic cells, can induce primary alloimmunity by both routes 1 and 2. Where an MHC-incompatible graft has been depleted of its content of dendritic cells, or happens to consist of tissue naturally devoid of such cells, it can only immunize via route 2, and in these circumstances its immunogenicity is comparable to minor system incompatibilities. This hypothesis does accommodate the fact that there is some strain variation in the results of retransplantation of kidney graft experiments. In certain donor/recipient combinations, the retransplanted kidneys are rejected (Hart *et al.*, 1980). The argument in these cases is that it results from immunization by route 2, and the important practical point here is that because route 2 is markedly less efficient than route 1, it would be predicted that very little immunosuppression would be needed to control route 2 responses. This prediction has been tested in the author's laboratory, and found to hold good (Lechler & Batchelor, 1982b).

The same basic experimental plan of retransplantation described earlier was used, except that a fully homozygous incompatible AUG strain kidney was retransplanted rather than the F_1. Retransplanted AUG grafts are rejected in AS recipients. Very high blood ureas are usually present by 10 days after grafting, and the rats show a median survival time of 22 days. A dose–response study of the amount of cyclophosphamide necessary to prevent the rejection of the retransplanted AUG kidneys, showed that 1·25 mg/kg for the first 2 weeks could prevent rejection. However, at least five times as much cyclophosphamide was required to produce an equivalent protection for a normal AUG kidney, i.e. one containing incompatible dendritic cells.

The hypothesis presented suggests a uniquely immunogenic role for dendritic cells and possibly other types of passenger cells in kidney allografts. By implication the same may be true of other types of graft. It therefore seemed important to attempt to isolate and characterize these cells. My co-worker, Dierdre Grennan, has recently developed a method of isolating these cells and we are in the process of studying them. It is already evident that there is more than one cell type carrying class II MHC antigens which can be liberated from rat kidneys by enzymes and gentle sieving, but one of them has at least some of the characteristics of dendritic cells.

Suppressor T cells and enhancement

Lastly, we should return to the problem of suppression in enhancement. The experimental systems we had previously used in our unsuccessful search for evidence of suppressor cells involved challenging rats injected with putative suppressors with a normal kidney or skin graft. However, if it is postulated that suppression develops gradually and only exerts a powerful effect during the maintenance phase of enhancement, this would be at a time when the graft was already depleted of incompatible passenger cells. Thus a passenger cell-depleted graft would be the proper challenge in a suppressor assay system. Failure to detect suppressor cells previously could be attributed to the strong immunogenicity of normal allografts with their content of dendritic cells.

The search for evidence of suppressor cells was renewed, using the following system (Batchelor, Phillips & Grennan, 1984). Firstly, an AS recipient is given an enhancement protocol and an $(AS \times AUG)F_1$ kidney allograft. After approximately 1 month, the recipient is well into the maintenance stage of enhancement and deeply unresponsive to AUG alloantigens. At this point the F_1 graft is replaced with an AUG strain kidney, which is 'parked' in the first recipient for a further month. During this time the passenger cells of AUG origin are lost and AS cells take their place. The AUG kidney is then retransplanted into a second, naive AS rat. As mentioned earlier, such grafts are rejected if no further action is taken. In the present experiments, the second AS recipient was also injected intravenously with spleen cells harvested from the first AS recipient. If suppressor cells in the first recipient were responsible for maintaining the survival of the AUG kidney, it should be possible to transfer them and modify the rejection of a graft already depleted of allogeneic passenger cells. The initial results show that spleen cells taken from the rats with enhanced kidneys do have a suppressive effect, whereas if no cells or normal AS spleen cells are injected, the AUG kidneys are rejected. It is concluded that suppressor cells are present in rats with enhanced kidneys. So far no studies have been done on the specificity of the suppression, but it has become evident that T cell-enriched suspensions, prepared by nylon wool filtration of cells from the spleens with suppressor activity, can also mediate suppression.

Conclusions and speculations

1   Immunological enhancement is an inappropriate phrase used to denote a series of complex events. For an understanding of the phenomenon, it is necessary to separate these events.

2   The prolonged survival of MHC-incompatible allografts in the maintenance stage of enhancement is due to at least two factors: (i) loss from the graft of highly immunogenic, MHC-incompatible dendritic cells, which are the only graft cells capable of direct activation of the recipient's T_H cells; (ii) the presence of suppressor T cells, the activity of which *may* not be discerned unless the graft has been depleted of highly immunogenic incompatible dendritic cells.

3   Probably the maintenance stage of enhancement is very similar in principle to the state of partial non-responsiveness towards organ grafts induced in animals and humans after variable but prolonged treatment with immunosuppressive drugs.

4   It is suggested that in passive enhancement, the critical function of enhancing antibody is to delay and minimize direct activation of the recipient's T_H by the MHC-incompatible dendritic cells of the allograft.

5   It is suggested that in active enhancement, the antigenic pretreatment regimen is effective because the inoculum contains minimal or no viable MHC-incompatible dendritic cells, but antigen in a form capable of activating suppressor cells.

Acknowledgment

Financial support for the work described was provided by the MRC.

References

Batchelor, J. R., Brent, L. & Kilshaw, P. J. (1977a) Absence of suppressor cells from rats bearing passively enhanced kidney allografts. *Nature (Lond.)*, **270**, 522.

Batchelor, J. R., Phillips, B. E. & Grennan, D. (1984) Suppressor cells and their role in the survival of immunologically enhanced rat kidney allografts. *Transplantation*, **37**, (in press).

Batchelor, J. R. & Welsh, K. I. (1976) Mechanisms of enhancement of kidney allograft survival. *Br. med. Bull.* **32**, 113.

Batchelor, J. R., Welsh, K. I. & Burgos, H. (1977b) Immunologic enhancement. *Transplant. Proc.* **9**, 931.

Batchelor, J. R., Welsh, K. I. & Burgos, H. (1978) Transplantation antigens *per se* are poor immunogens within a species. *Nature (Lond.)*, **273**, 54.

Batchelor, J. R., Welsh, K. I., Maynard, A. & Burgos, H. (1979) Failure of long surviving, passively enhanced kidney allografts to provoke T-dependent alloimmunity. *J. exp. Med.* **150**, 455.

Bowen, J. E., Batchelor, J. R., French, M. E., Burgos, H. & Fabre, J. W. (1974) Failure of adoptive immunization or parabiosis with hyperimmune syngeneic partners to abrogate long-term enhancement of rat kidney allografts. *Transplantation*, **18**, 322.

Fabre, J. W. & Morris, P. J. (1972) The mechanism of specific immunosuppression of renal allografts rejection by donor strain blood. *Transplantation*, **14**, 634.

Fine, R. N., Batchelor, J. R., French, M. E. & Shumak, K. H. (1973) The uptake of ^{125}I-labelled rat alloantibody and its loss after combination with antigen. *Transplantation*, **16**, 641.

French, M. E. & Batchelor, J. R. (1969) Immunological enhancement of rat kidney grafts. *Lancet*, **ii**, 1103.

French, M. E., Batchelor, J. R. & Watts, H. G. (1971) The capacity of lymphocytes from rats bearing enhanced kidney allografts to mount graft-versus-host reactions. *Transplantation*, **12**, 45.

Gorer, P. A. (1961) The antigenic structure of tumors. *Adv. Immunol.* **1**, 345.

Hart, D. N. J., Winnearls, C. G. & Fabre, J. W. (1980) Graft adaptation: studies on possible mechanisms in long-term surviving rat renal allografts. *Transplantation*, **30**, 73.

Kaliss, N. (1958) Immunological enhancement of tumor homografts in mice: a review. *Cancer Res.* **18**, 992.

Kilshaw, P. J. & Brent, L. (1977) Further studies on suppressor T cells in mice unresponsive to H-2 incompatible skin grafts. *Transplant. Proc.* **9**, 717.

Lechler, R. I. & Batchelor, J. R. (1982a) Restoration of immunogenicity to passenger cell-depleted kidney allografts by the addition of donor strain dendritic cells. *J. Exp. Med.* **155**, 31.

Lechler, R. I. & Batchelor, J. R. (1982b) Immunogenicity of retransplanted rat kidney allografts. *J. exp. Med.* **156**, 1835.

Lee, S. (1967) An improved technique of renal transplantation in the rat. *Surgery*, **61**, 771.

Mason, D. W., Pugh, C. W. & Webb, M. (1981) The rat mixed lymphocyte reaction: roles of a dendritic cell in intestinal lymph and T cell subsets defined by monoclonal antibodies. *Immunology*, **44**, 75.

Steinmann, R. M. & Nussenzweig, M. C. (1980) Dendritic cells: features and functions. *Immunol. Rev.* **53**, 127.

Welsh, K. I., Burgos, H. & Batchelor, J. R. (1977) The immune response to allogeneic rat platelets; Ag-B antigens in matrix form lacking Ia. *Eur. J. Immunol.* **7**, 267.

Chapter 5
Recognition of minor transplantation antigens: the role of H-2 and other Ir genes

Elizabeth Simpson

Transplantation Biology Section, Clinical Research Centre, Watford Road, Harrow, Middlesex HA1 3UJ.

Summary. Minor transplantation antigens are recognized by T cells in the context of self major histocompatibility complex (MHC) antigens. Immune responses to minor histocompatibility (H) antigens are regulated by both class I and class II MHC gene products, and in addition by Ir genes outside the MHC. Some of these non-MHC Ir genes have been mapped with respect to responses to the minor H antigen, H-Y, but their identity and mode of action are not yet understood. Immune responses to minor H antigens include graft rejection, generation of MHC-restricted cytotoxic T cell responses during *in vitro* mixed lymphocyte culture (MLC), antigen-specific proliferation in MLC, host-versus-graft reaction and delayed-type hypersensitivity *in vivo*.

The biological role of syngeneic minor H antigens is very poorly understood. It has been proposed that they may play a role in differentiation during embryogenesis. The hypothesis that the male-specific minor H antigen H-Y plays this role during primary sex determination has been explored by H-Y typing a series of karyotypically abnormal mice with paradoxical sex phenotypes.

Introduction

In mice, H-2 are clearly the strongest transplantation antigens, but from a very early stage in the experiments which defined them, it was clear that they were not the sole polymorphic alloantigens which could stimulate graft rejection (Klein, 1975). These other, non-H-2 transplantation antigens were called minor transplantation antigens, or, in the words of Don Bailey, H non-2 antigens. Incompatibilities at multiple minor loci between H-2-matched strains gave rise to fairly rapid graft rejection (Bailey, 1971a). However, when the influence of individual loci were examined in isolation, using minor H congenic mouse strains, graft rejection times were generally much longer, exemplifying the 'weak' nature of individual antigens (Bailey, 1975, 1981).

Shortly after the discovery that self H-2 molecules were vitally important for the recognition of extrinsic antigens such as viruses and haptens by T cells (Zinkernagel & Doherty, 1974; Shearer, 1974), it was realized that the recognition of minor H alloantigens was governed by the same rules of H-2 restriction. Initially these findings were made for cytotoxic T cell responses to multiple minor H antigens (Bevan, 1975) and the single minor H antigen H-Y (Gordon, Simpson & Samelson, 1975), but subsequently this has been found for a number of isolated minor H antigens (Wettstein & Frelinger, 1980; Mobraaten, Bailey & Sarjent, unpublished; Loveland, in preparation).

The target cell specificity of cytotoxic T cell responses to minor H antigens indicates that each antigen is recognized in the context of a self class I (K or D) H-2 molecule. The manner of recognition of the two presumably associated moieties, self H-2 K or D on the one hand and allogeneic minor H antigen on the other, is still not understood. However, certain H-2 molecules are preferentially employed in H-2-restricted recognition by cytotoxic cells (e.g. in H-2^b mice, H-Y is always restricted to D^b, and not K^b, in the cytotoxic T cell response) and thus class I H-2 genes are one type of Ir gene controlling these responses.

Helper T cells are also needed during the generation of minor H specific cytotoxic T cells (Simon *et al.*, 1981; Tomonari, submitted; Gascoigne, 1983) and these, unlike cytotoxic cells, are restricted by class II self H-2 molecules. In this sense class II genes are also Ir genes.

The ability to dissect out and map the influence of Ir genes depends on examining an antigen to which immune responsiveness is variable in a genetically determined way. The antigen should induce responses in some inbred mouse strains but not others. The male-specific antigen, H-Y, is such an example, and a detailed analysis of several T cell responses to H-Y, and the genetics of these responses, has led us to the conclusion that not only H-2 but also non-H-2 genes can act as Ir genes. Furthermore, at least some non-H-2 Ir genes seem to interact with H-2 Ir genes to determine responsiveness. This again focuses attention on the pivotal importance of H-2 genes in the control of immune responsiveness.

H-Y was originally discovered as a transplantation antigen by Eichwald & Silmser (1955) who found that female mice of certain strains would reject syngeneic male skin grafts. Since the only difference between males and females of the same inbred strain is the possession of the Y chromosome by the male, these data were interpreted by Hauschka (1955) and Snell (1956) as evidence for the presence of a minor histocompatibility (H) locus on the Y chromosome, hence the name, H-Y.

Since that time, attempts to identify polymorphism of the H-Y antigen expressed by mice from many different sources, including wild mice, have produced no evidence of H-Y alleles (Gasser & Silvers, 1972; Gasser, Silvers & Wachtel, 1974; Simpson *et al.*, 1979; Johnson, 1982; Mintz & Silvers, 1983) and this has made it very difficult to map the structural gene for H-Y with certainty. All the data are consistent with it being located on the Y chromosome, but it cannot yet be excluded that a controlling gene is on the Y chromosome, with the structural gene on an autosome or the X chromosome. The biochemical nature of the H-Y antigen is not yet determined. It is assumed to be a cell surface molecule, because of its functional association with MHC class I and II molecules (see above). A male-specific antigen identified serologically was originally assumed to be the same as H-Y, but this now seems unlikely in view of discordant typing of XO mice, which are H-Y-negative yet serologically positive (Melvold *et al.*, 1977; Engel, Klemme & Ebrecht, 1981; Simpson, McClaren & Chandler, 1982). It has been proposed that the serologically defined male antigen be named SDM (Silvers, Gasser & Eicher, 1982).

In this paper we shall therefore concentrate on T cell responses to H-Y. Two of these have already been mentioned, namely, graft rejection and the generation of cytotoxic T cells. In addition, two further *in vivo* responses have been identified, delayed-type hypersensitivity (DTH) and host-versus-graft (HvG) responses. The DTH response correlates extremely well with the skin graft rejection response (Liew & Simpson, 1980; Greene, Benacerraf & Dorf, 1980), and is one of the pieces of evidence that skin graft rejection is mediated by Ly-1$^+$2$^-$ DTH T cells restricted by class II MHC antigens, rather than Ly-1$^+$2$^+$ cytotoxic T cells restricted by class I MHC antigens. The HvG response may be the *in vivo* correlate of Ly-1$^+$ T helper cells necessary for the induction of the cytotoxic T cell response (Pole & Simpson, 1983). In addition to the cytotoxic T cell response generated in secondary MLC, *in vitro* T cell proliferative responses to H-Y can be detected and used to type mice for the presence of H-Y. Proliferative responses to H-Y are most clearly shown by cloned T cells and two types have been isolated: type one is restricted by class I MHC antigens, and generally this type is IL-2-dependent and has cytotoxic function (von Boehmer *et al.*, 1979; Tomonari, 1983a; Simpson *et al.*, 1984); type two is class II MHC-restricted, will proliferate to H-Y on appropriate cells in the absence of IL-2, and is not cytotoxic, but can be shown to have helper function *in vitro* and *in vivo* (Tomonari 1983a, and submitted).

The influence of class I and II MHC genes on anti-H-Y responses

Initial observations on H-2 control of both graft rejection and cytotoxic responses to H-Y indicated that mice with the H-2^b haplotype were particularly good responders, and could be distinguished from mice of a large number of other haplotypes, including H-2^k, H-2^d, H-2^s, H-2^f, H-2^r, H-2^m, H-2^q (Bailey, 1971b; Gordon & Simpson, 1977; Hurme et al., 1978a, b; Simpson, 1982). Only H-2^b females, or intra H-2^b recombinants having the K + I regions of the H-2^b haplotype can reject primary H-Y-incompatible skin grafts, although certain strains of some other H-2 haplotypes can be induced by previous subcutaneous (s.c.) (into the footpad) immunization to reject syngeneic male grafts in a second set fashion (Simpson et al., 1983a). Females of all the H-2^b strains examined (C57BL/10, C57BL/6, A.BY, C3H.SW, BALB.B) will make cytotoxic T cell responses to H-Y in secondary MLC, following a previous intraperitoneal (i.p.) or intravenous (i.v.) immunization with syngeneic male cells (Table 5.1). In contrast, non-H-2^b females will not make anti-H-Y responses in MLC after i.p. or i.v. immunization in vivo (Table 5.1). However, some but not all strains of at least the H-2^k, H-2^d and H-2^s haplotypes can be induced to respond in MLC in vitro if their in vivo immunization is made subcutaneously into the footpad (fp) (see next section).

The difference in anti-H-Y reactivity between H-2^b and other H-2 haplotypes lies principally in the H-2 I region. Possession of the H-2 I-A^b allele allows for readily elicited I-A^b restricted helper cell responses to H-Y, and these are required for generation of cytotoxic responses (Hurme et al., 1977; Michaelides et al., 1981) and probably also for graft rejection/DTH responses. It is clear however that H-Y-specific helper cells can under appropriate immunization conditions be generated in H-2^k mice, where they can be H-2 I-A^k and/or H-2 I-E^k restricted (Brenan & Müllbacher, 1981). From the responsiveness of some H-2^d and H-2^s strains following fp immunization (Fierz et al., 1982a, b) it is assumed that H-2 I^d- and H-2 I^s-restricted helper cells can likewise be generated. It is unclear why I-A^b-restricted H-Y-specific helper cell responses are so readily triggered in comparison with those of other haplotypes. It is possible that the balance of helper and suppressor cells is different in H-2^b mice and favours helpers, but there is abundant evidence that H-2^b mice also possess H-Y-specific suppressors (Simpson et al., 1981a).

When H-2^b homozygous mice respond to H-Y, their cytotoxic T cells are restricted to D^b and never to K^b (both are class I MHC antigens) (Table 5.1). Thus it could be said that D^b is a 'permissive' allele for H-Y, whilst K^b is 'not permissive'. When H-2 heterozygous female mice with one H-2^b (responder) parent and one non-H-2^b (non-responder) parent are examined for responsiveness to H-Y, it is found that cytotoxic responses can be readily generated to male cells of either parental type

Table 5.1. Influence of H-2 class I and class II genes on responsiveness to H-Y

Mouse strain	H-2 haplotypes	Primary graft rejection of syngeneic or semisyngeneic skin	Cytotoxicity* and restriction element	
C57BL/10	b			
C57BL/6				
A.BY		$+$	$+$	H-2D^b
C3H.SW				
BALB.B				
B10.BR	k			
B10.D2	d			
B10.S	s	$-$	$-$	
B10.RIII	r			
B10.M	f			
(B10 × B10.BR)F$_1$	b × k	F$_1$$^\delta$+	$+$	H-2D^k‡
		B10.BR$^\delta$+	$+$	H-2D^k§
		B10$^\delta$±†	$+$	H-2D^b¶
(B10 × B10.D2)F$_1$	b × d	F$_1$$^\delta$+	$+$	H-2D^b‡
		B10.D2$^\delta$+	$+$	H-2K^d§
		B10$^\delta$+	$+$	H-2D^b¶
(B10 × B10.S)F$_1$	b × s	F$_1$$^\delta$+	$+$	H-2D^s‡
		B10.S$^\delta$+	$+$	H-2D^s§
		B10$^\delta$+	$+$	H-2D^b¶

* Following i.p. *in vivo* immunization and secondary restimulation *in vitro* in MLC.
† Some but not all grafts rejected. (+ All grafts rejected.)
‡ Following immunization and restimulation with F$_1$ male cells.
§ Following immunization and restimulation with P$_1$ male cells.
¶ Following immunization and restimulation with P$_2$ male cells.
Data summarized from Gordon *et al.* (1975), Gordon & Simpson (1977), Simpson & Gordon (1977), Gordon *et al.* (1977), Brenan *et al.* (1981), Müllbacher *et al.* (1981) and Chandler (unpublished).

following i.p. or i.v. immunization (Gordon, Samelson & Simpson, 1977). In general, immunization *in vivo* and restimulation *in vitro* with F_1 hybrid male cells will generate a response to H-Y in association with only one parental type (the 'preferred parent'), but when both immunization and restimulation are carried out with the same homozygous parental cells, the cytotoxic response will be restricted to the class I MHC antigens of the parental cells used (Table 5.1). In this way, H-Y-specific responses restricted to the H-2 type of the non-responder parent can readily be generated. This shows that non responsiveness, or inability to respond after i.p. or i.v. *in vivo* immunization in non-H-2^b strains is not due to lack of H-Y antigen or to their possession of 'non-permissive" class I alleles. Class I MHC antigens of all haplotypes examined have been found capable of restricting H-Y-specific cytotoxic T cells. In general, either the H-2K allele (e.g. H-2K^d) or the H-2D allele (e.g. H-2D^b, H-2D^k, H-2D^s, H-2D^q) of any one haplotype is permissive, whilst the other is not and the restriction element for each haplotype is the same, whether the response is generated in H-2 heterozygotes (Table 5.1) or in homozygotes (Tables 5.1, 5.2).

In summary, the influences of H-2 Ir genes on H-Y responsiveness are two-fold. First, class I gene products restrict cytotoxic T cells and some are permissive (D^b, K^d, D^k, D^s, D^q) whilst others are non-permissive (K^b, D^d, K^s, K^q). Secondly, class II gene products restrict helper cells which are necessary for generating the cytotoxic response. I-A^b is not the only permissive allele, but in order to demonstrate others, for example I-A^k and I-E^k, it is necessary to resort to particular routes of immunization (fp).

The influence of non-H-2 Ir genes on anti-H-Y responses

The first indication that non-H-2 Ir genes were involved in regulating anti-H-Y responses came from the observation that certain H-2^k, H-2^d and H-2^s strains, but not all, could be induced to make good cytotoxic responses after footpad immunization (Fierz *et al.*, 1982a). These results are summarized in Table 5.2(a). From these it is also apparent that there is an interaction between the non-H-2 Ir genes and the H-2 haplotype. Take, for example, the response pattern of H-2^d and H-2^k mice: on a BALB background, H-2^d are non-responders (BALB/c), whilst H-2^k are responders (BALB.K). In contrast, H-2^d on the B10 background (B10.D2) respond, whilst H-2^k (B10.BR) do not. Thus, responsiveness is determined by an interaction between H-2 and non-H-2 'background' genes, and particular constellations of each are necessary to ensure responsiveness; neither H-2 nor non-H-2 genes alone determine responsiveness but together they do. The manner of their proposed interaction is speculative until the nature of the non-H-2 Ir genes for H-Y responsiveness is determined. As a first step to this, studies were undertaken to map the non-H-2 genes involved in determining responsiveness in H-2^d and H-2^k mice.

Two approaches were used, one by comparing the responses of Igh congenic pairs of mouse strains, thus examining the role of the Igh locus (Farmer, Fierz & Simpson, 1983), and secondly by determining the strain distribution pattern (SDP) of anti-H-Y responsiveness amongst sets of recombinant inbred (RI) strains for which SDP of many genes of known

Table 5.2. Influence of non-H-2 genes on cytotoxic T cell responses to H-Y

Strain	H-2 haplotype	Responsiveness*
(a) CBA/H	k	+
C3H/He		±
BALB.K		+
C58/J		±
Ce/J		−
AKR		−
B10.BR		−
B10.D2	d	+
B6.C H-2^d		+
BALB/c		−
DBA/2		−
A.SW	s	−
B10.S		+

(b)	H-2	Igh	
CBA	k	j	+
CB.20	k	b	+
BALB/c	d	a	−
BALB.B20	d	b	−

* +, >80% mice of this strain respond. ±, 30–80% mice of this strain respond. −, 0% mice of this strain respond.

Data summarized from Fierz et al. (1982a, b), Farmer et al. (1983).

location are available (Fierz *et al.*, 1982b). By comparing SDP of the unknown gene with those of the known genes, it is usually possible to assign the unknown gene to a chromosomal location (Bailey, 1981).

Table 5.2(b) summarizes the results using two sets of Igh congenic pairs to determine the possible influence of the Igh locus. It is clear that there is none, in that substitution of the Igh^a allele present in the non-responder BALB/c strain into the responder CBA (Igh^j) strain does not alter responsiveness, and likewise, substitution of the Igh^b allele present in the B10.D2 responder strain into the non-responder BALB/c (Igh^a) strain does not affect responsiveness.

The use of RI strains has been much more informative (Fierz *et al.*, 1982b); the BXD strains derived from the C57BL/6 strain (B10.D2 and B6.C H-2^d are responders to H-Y) and the DBA/2 strain (non-responder to H-Y) were examined, restricting the analysis to the H-2^d strains, since it is only amongst non-H-2^b strains that the influence of non-H-2 Ir genes is apparent (compare Tables 5.1 and 5.2). Approximately half a dozen female mice of each H-2^d BXD RI strain were immunized subcutaneously in the footpad with syngeneic male cells, and the number of mice of each strain making an H-Y-specific response on subsequent restimulation of MLC was determined. For this analysis, each strain was then designated as a responder if any of its females responded to H-Y, or as a non-responder if none did. Since the responses were somewhat variable (as is often the case with non-H-2^b mice: see Fierz *et al.*, 1982a, and Table 5.2), our assignment of responder/non-responder status was open to a degree of doubt, since 'false negatives' could easily place a potential responder strain into a non-responder category. However, initial analysis of the SDP of responsiveness determined in this way showed an almost complete correlation with the SDP of the β_2-microblobulin (β_2m) gene on chromosome 2. If then a chi-squared analysis was done, putting together the cytotoxicity results of all the mice tested, and comparing responsiveness/non-responsiveness with the a and the b allele of β_2m for which this RI set has segregated, it is clear, as shown in Table 5.3, that there is a significant association of responsiveness with the β_2m^b allele (12/28 responders) and of non-responsiveness with the β_2m^a allele (32/33 non-responders). This association is significant ($P < 0.0005$), and maps this non-H-2 Ir gene for H-Y responsiveness at or closely linked to β_2m. Subsequently we have examined a pair of H-2^d β_2m/H-3 congenic mouse strains for responsiveness to H-Y, but have found both strains, regardless of β_2m/H-3 allele, to be responders to H-Y (Farmer, Wettstein & Simpson, unpublished). This result would suggest that the H-Y Ir gene for responsiveness in H-2^d mice is closely linked to β_2m, but is not β_2m itself. It is likely, however, that this β_2m-linked gene is not the only non-H-2 gene affecting responsiveness in H-2^d mice, since comparison of B10.D2 and B6.C-H-2^d, which differ only in the non-H-2 genes at which B10 and B6 differ, do not give the same proportion of responders to H-Y (Fierz *et al.*, 1982b). B10.D2 respond more often than do B6.C H-2^d, but the quantification of this sort of effect would take such large numbers of mice, tested under invariant conditions, that the whole exercise would hardly seem justified. In order to pursue the question of degree of responsiveness, other approaches will be necessary.

Table 5.3. H-Y responsiveness in H-2^d BXD RI strains

	+	−	
β_2m^b	12	16	
			$P = <0.0005$
β_2m^a	1	3	

Summarized from Fierz *et al.* (1982b).

The use of RI strains to map the non-H-2 genes for H-2^k strains has not produced the same relatively clear-cut results as the BXD strains. The BXH RI strains, derived from the C57BL/6 strain (B10.BR is a non-responder) and the C3H/He strain (C3H is a responder) comprise six H-2^k strains and seven H-2^b strains. As already mentioned, only the H-2^k strains are potentially informative, so only these were tested. Their SDP of anti-H-Y responsiveness implicated three genes, one on chromosome 1 at or close to *Lsh* and two on chromosome 12 (one at or close to rRNA-Ae and the other to Epa; Farmer, 1983). Because of the small number of strains involved, the analysis is limited but it is clear that neither the Igh locus is involved nor a β_2m-linked locus, thus confirming the findings with the Igh congenics (Table 5.2b) and the strain distribution pattern of responsiveness amongst inbred laboratory mouse strains (Table 5.2a). Thus we may expect that for each H-2 haplotype examined, a different locus (or loci) will be found, acting as non-H-2 H-Y Ir gene(s). Again, the prospect of systematically tracking these down, when one takes into account the somewhat variable anti-H-Y cytotoxic T cell responsiveness of non-H-2^b mice, does not appeal using the methods applied so far, so new approaches will be necessary.

The use of graft rejection, cytotoxic T cells and cloned T cells to H-Y type mice with genetic or developmental abnormalities

It was proposed several years ago that H-Y in particular, and perhaps minor H antigens in general, might act as differentiation signals during embryogenesis (Wachtel *et al.*, 1975; Ohno, 1977). These antigens were deemed ideally situated for this function, in being cell surface molecules anchored in the surface membrane by MHC molecules. This much was implied by the target cell specificity of anti minor H cytotoxic T cells (Gordon, Simpson & Samelson, 1975; Bevan, 1975). Most of the H-Y arguments were made for the serologically detected male antigen (SDM, see above) which was assumed to be H-Y, but which now appears to be different from H-Y. Nevertheless, discussion of H-Y as a possible trigger for the differentiation of testis from the gonadal anlage has continued, and this discussion has been sharpened recently by the discovery of several different situations which give rise to sex reversal in mice, i.e. XX individuals which paradoxically can develop into males, and XY individuals which paradoxically develop into females.

The H-Y typing of such mice is of obvious interest, since it would be expected to throw light on whether the presence of H-Y antigen was invariably associated with testis formation. However, H-Y typing using the graft rejection or the cytotoxic T cell response can be done most easily in inbred mice, and preferably those either homozygous or heterozygous for H-2^b. Given these conditions, mice can be typed as H-Y-positive if (i) they fail to make anti-H-Y responses, (ii) their cells serve as targets for anti-H-Y cytotoxic T cell responses. Likewise, mice can be typed as H-Y-negative if (i) they make anti-H-Y responses, (ii) their cells do not serve as targets for anti-H-Y cytotoxic T cells. These criteria have been used to H-Y type various mice (Melvold *et al.*, 1977; Johnson *et al.*, 1983; Simpson *et al.*, 1981b, 1982, 1983b, 1984). In situations where the genetic or developmental abnormality under scrutiny was present in a non-inbred stock, it was sometimes possible to cross the mice carrying the abnormality with inbred H-2^b mice, and use the heterozygotes as responders to homozygous H-2^b male tissue, or as targets for H-2^b-restricted killer cells (Simpson *et al.*, 1981b, 1982, 1984).

The results of these studies are summarized in Table 5.4, and show that H-Y is not invariably associated with testis formation, in that XY females, which arise by back-crossing the Y chromosome from various wild mouse strains on to the C57BL/6 background, are H-Y-positive, but these mice have ovaries and normal female genitalia (Eicher *et al.*, 1982; Johnson *et al.*, 1983; Simpson *et al.*, 1983b). The other finding of note is that XO mice can develop as females (as most do), or more rarely as males (one reported case), but although both are H-Y-negative, both types are reported SDM-positive (Melvold *et al.*, 1977; Engel *et al.*, 1981; Simpson *et al.*, 1982).

Recently we have been investigating the H-Y status of XX *Sxr* mice (Cattanach, Pollard & Hawkes, 1971), which generally develop as males which are H-Y-positive (Simpson *et al.*, 1981), but which by genetic manipulation of the X inactivation process can develop as females (McLaren & Monk, 1982). The typing of these mice was initially done with cytotoxic T cells, either H-2^k- or H-2^b-restricted, since the non-inbred mouse stocks used to generate the mice under test were either H-2^b

Table 5.4. H-Y and SDM typing of normal and karyotypically abnormal mice of various types

Phenotypic sex	Sex chromosome karyotype	H-Y	SDM	References
Female	XX	−	−	Eichwald & Silmser (1955) Goldberg *et al.* (1972)
Male	XY	+	+	Gordon, Samelson & Simpson (1975)
Female	XO	−	+	Engel *et al.* (1981) Simpson *et al.* (1980)
Male	XO	−	+	Melvold *et al.* (1977)
Male	XX*Sxr*	+	+	Cattenach *et al.* (1971) Bennett *et al.* (1977) Simpson *et al.* (1981b)
Male	T(16; X)16HX	+	NT	McLaren & Monk (1982) Simpson *et al.* (1984)
Female	T(16; X)16HX	+	NT	This paper
Female	XY^{POS}	+	NT	Johnson *et al.* (1983)
Female	XY^{ORB}	+	NT	Simpson *et al.* (1983b)
Hermaphrodite	XY^{POS}	+	NT	
Hermaphrodite	XY^{ORB}	+	NT	

Summarized from Simpson *et al.* (1983b, 1984).

or H-2^k (mostly H-2^k homozygotes, although a few H-2^b homozygotes and k × b heterozygotes were found). Since the mice were not inbred, and it was not possible to study their developmental abnormalities by making heterozygotes with an inbred mouse strain, the H-Y typing was confined to using their cells as targets for H-Y-specific T cells, and as stimulator cells for H-Y-specific T cell clones (Tomonari, 1983a, and in preparation). The clones were used in proliferative assays, which have been shown to be extremely sensitive in detecting even small numbers of H-Y-positive cells in a mixed population of normal XX and XY cells (Chandler, Burgoyne & Simpson, in preparation). The class I-restricted H-Y-specific clones 10-2

Table 5.5. Proliferative responses of H-Y-specific T cell clones

Stimulating cells (KID)		Clone (origin and restriction specificity)		
		2-1-1(B6.I-A^b)	10-2(B6.D^b)	C-3(C3H, D^k)
None		199	541	
C57BL/6♂	bbb	**26,637**	**241,455**	
C57BL/6♀	bbb	389	1988	
B10.A(5R)♂	bbd	**31,085**	3558†	
B10.A(4R)♂	kkb	219		
B10.A(2R)♂	kkb		**270,175**	
bm12♂	bb*b	177	**172,956‡**	
bm14♂	bbb*		5025	
CBA♂	kkk			**108,970**
CBA♀	kkk			557
C3H.OH♂	ddk			**176,428**
B10.A♂	kkd			648

† Data from a separate experiment in which the stimulation by C57BL/6♂ was 65,434, and medium only was 1575.

‡ From a separate experiment in which addition of C57BL/6♂ gave 287,737 c.p.m., and medium alone gave 1910.

Cells from each clone were placed in 100 μl medium at 10^4 per well in flat-bottomed wells of microtitre places. In control wells (no stimulating cells) an additional 100 μl medium alone was added for clone 2-1-1, while for clones 10-2 and C-3 100 μl medium and 50 μl rat concanavalin A (Con A) supernatant were added. Fifty microlitres of Con A supernatant was added to all wells containing 10-2 and C-3 cells. Eight hundred thousand irradiated, RBC-depleted spleen cells per well were added to triplicate wells, using as donors of spleen cells the mouse strains shown. After 72 hr (clone 2-1-1), 96 hr (clone 10-2) or 120 hr (clone C-3), the wells were pulsed with [^{3}H]-thymidine, 1 μCi/well and harvested 6–8 hr later.

Data taken from Tomonari (1983a, and in preparation).

(D^b-restricted) and C-3 (D^k-restricted) were stimulated by irradiated spleen cells from control and test mice in the presence of IL-2, on which they are dependent, whilst the class II-restricted clone 2-1 ($I-A^b$-restricted) was similarly stimulated, but in the absence of IL-2. Table 5.5 shows experimental data which establish the restriction specificity of these clones.

Table 5.6 gives some data from an experiment in which XX female, XY male and XX *Sxr* male and female mice were typed for H-2 and H-Y by cytotoxic T cells, and for H-Y by the proliferative responses of the H-Y-specific T cell clones. The results of each mode of typing for H-Y are

Table 5.6. H-Y typing by CML and proliferation of H-Y-specific clones of normal mice, and of mice of both sex phenotypes carrying *Sxr*

Cells added from mouse	Proliferation of H-Y-specific clone (restriction specificity)			CML typing with	
	C-3(D^k)	10-2(D^b)	2-1($I-A^b$)	anti-H-Y $H-2^k$	anti-H-Y $H-2^b$
None	1026	301	765		
30 XX♀	2174	1078	197	0·9	1·1
32	929	1312	489	−1·2	2·0
33	1487	552	245	−14·4	−7·7
34	591	649	3932	3·0	1·7
4 XX *Sxr*♀	**26,406**	651	3252	**20·0**	8·5
13	**58,269**	379	3086	**30·6**	6·4
35	**66,208**	828	518	**26·4**	8·4
36	**42,014**	1531	2526	**23·0**	−1·1
37	**46,783**	586	2053	**23·3**	5·8
38	**64,640**	1255	1160	**29·4**	2·0
39	1904	1648	1685	1·3	1·9
40	**61,249**	1613	4149	**25·2**	3·1
41	**47,145**	778	7653	**25·8**	6·2
42 XX *Sxr*♂	**82,529**	1229	704	ND	ND
43	**40,797**	341	225	ND	ND
47	899	**22,400**	ND	−0·7	**12·4**
31 XY♂	549	**32,610**	**30,472**	−3·7	**29·4**
45	**3178**	1451	579	**29·3**	2·7
46	**12,092**	635	30	**16·9**	−1·1

For method of proliferation see legend for Table 5.5
CML: % cytotoxicity at A:T 10:1 from 12 point regression analysis.

concordant, and indicate that all but one of the XX *Sxr* females were H-Y-positive. Since all these females were fertile (McLaren & Monk, 1982), this result indicates that the presence of H-Y antigen is not inconsistent with formation of the ovary and female genitalia and with normal reproductive function.

The H-Y-negative XX *Sxr* female is of interest. One possible explanation of the negative finding could be that only a very small proportion of her spleen cells are H-Y-positive, and that these fall below the level at which they can be detected by the assays used. If this were the case, then this individual is clearly different from the other XX *Sxr* females who showed no evidence from the cytotoxic typing of a lower proportion of H-Y-positive spleen cells than the XY control males. The variation in the level of proliferative responses is probably due to variation of the day at which peak responses are elicited by spleen cells from the different mice tested. Experiments using inbred mouse strains of a single haplotype ($H-2^k$) on several different backgrounds indicate that this timing effect may be controlled by non-H-2 genes (Tomonari, unpublished). Another possible explanation of the negative H-Y typing of mouse number 39 (and this has been confirmed in another experiment, which included a time course using the C-3 clone) is that the H-Y gene has been lost from the *Sxr* segment carried by this female. Since she is fertile, this explanation is testable and is currently under investigation (for recent results see McClaren *et al.*, 1984). Since the *Sxr* segment carries H-Y and a testis determining gene, separation of the two would prove that they were not the same, and this clearly has interesting biological implications.

A comparison of H-Y with other minor H antigens

Chromosomal mapping has placed other minor H antigens on almost every autosome, i.e. they are distributed throughout the genome (Bailey, 1975, 1981). They all share the property of stimulating skin allograft rejection and many of them have also been shown to elicit H-2-restricted cytotoxic T cell responses of the type described for H-Y. H-2 Ir gene control for these is clear (Wettstein & Frelinger, 1980) but so far no non-H-2 Ir genes for these responses have been reported, although non-H-2 Ir genes which influence H-2-restricted cytotoxic T cell responses to haptens coupled to syngeneic cells have been described (Fujiwara & Shearer, 1981). Host-versus-graft (HvG) responses have also been described to minor H antigens (Johnson, Bailey & Mobraaten, 1981) and these are Lyt-1^+2^--mediated. T cell responses (Pole & Simpson, 1983). In the case of anti-H-Y HvG responses, both H-2 and non-H-2 Ir genes are involved (Pole & Simpson, 1983).

Thus H-Y and the many other minor transplantation antigens have in common the propensity to stimulate T cells, and to be recognized by T cells in the context of self class I and class II MHC molecules. This implies that they too are membrane-bound molecules, although the possibility cannot be excluded that they are molecules which otherwise alter or interfere with the conformation of MHC molecules, without themselves being components of the cell membrane. Our knowledge of the structure of the T cell receptor should soon give insight into this question, as would isolation of the structural genes for the minor H antigens themselves.

From studies of immunological response to minor H antigens in the mouse, it is clear that they are intimately associated with H-2 and perhaps other cell surface molecules (e.g. the non-H-2 Ir gene products). Their biological properties as self determinants, as opposed to alloantigens, are obscure, but they would be well placed to be involved in cell–cell recognition during embryogenesis and perhaps in growth and differentiation processes throughout life. Further investigation of this area will require knowledge of the structure of the minor H antigens themselves, and of the genomic structural and control elements. We have been led into this area by studies of T cells and of H-2, the key components of self–non-self discrimination during adult life.

Acknowledgments

I would like to thank Sir Peter Medawar for his constant help and encouragement over the last 15 years, during which time the work of our laboratory on immune responses to weak antigens, H-Y in particular, has been pursued. I would like to thank my colleagues over the years, who have collaborated with me in the published H-Y work cited and reviewed here, namely, Robert Gordon, Larry Samelson, Mikko Hurme, Colin Hetherington, Takeshi Matsunaga, David Benjamin, Carolyn Brunner, Arno Müllbacher, Mary Brenan, Walter Fierz, David Pole and Eva Eicher. I also thank my colleagues Phillip Chandler, Bruce Loveland, Kyuhei Tomonari and Anne McLaren for permission to include discussion of some of our current collaborative work which has not yet been published.

References

Bailey, D. W. (1971a) Cumulative or independent effect. *Transplantation*, **11**, 419.

Bailey, D. W. (1971b) Allelic forms of a gene controlling the female immune response to the male antigen in mice. *Transplantation*, **11**, 426.

Bailey, D. W. (1975) Genetics of histocompatibility in mice. I. New loci and congenic lines. *Immunogenetics*, **2**, 249.

Bailey, D. W. (1981) Recombinant inbred strains and bilinneal congenic strains. In: *The Mouse in Biomedical Research*, Vol. 1 (eds Foster, Small and Fox). Academic Press.

Bennett, D., Mathieson, B. J., Scheid, M., Yanagisawa, K., Boyse, E. A., Wachtel, S. & Cattanach, B. M. (1977) Serological evidence for H-Y antigen in *Sxr* sex-reversed phenotypic males. *Nature (Lond.)*, **265**, 255.

Bevan, M. J. (1975) The major histocompatibility complex determines susceptibility to cytotoxic T cells directed against minor histocompatibility antigens. *J. exp. Med.* **142**, 1349.

Brenan, M. & Müllbacher, A. (1981) Analysis of H-2 determinants recognized during the induction of H-Y immune cytotoxic T cells by monoclonal antibodies *in vitro*. *J. exp. Med.* **154**, 563.

Brenan, M., Simpson, E. & Müllbacher, A. (1981) Analysis of haplotype preference in the cytotoxic T cell response to H-Y. *Immunogenetics*, **13**, 133.

Cattanach, B. M., Pollard, C. E. & Hawkes, S. G. (1971) Sex reversed mice: XX and XO moles. *Cytogenetics*, **10**, 318.

Eicher, E. M., Washburn, L. L., Whitney, J. B. III & Morrow, K. E. (1982) *Mus poschiavinus* Y chromosome in the C57BL/6J murine genome causes sex reversal. *Science*, 217, 535.

Eichwald, E. J. & Silmser, C. R. (1955) Untitled communication. *Transplant. Bull.* **2**, 148.

Engel, W., Klemme, B. & Ebrecht, A. (1981) Serological evidence for H-Y antigen in XO female mice. *Human Genet.* **57**, 68.

Farmer, G. A. (1983) Immune response gene control of the cytotoxic T-cell response to the H-Y antigen. *PhD Thesis*, Glasgow University.

Farmer, G. A., Fierz, W. & Simpson, E. (1983) The effect of the immunoglobulin heavy chain locus on the anti H-Y cytotoxic T-cell response in mice. *Transplant. Proc.* **15**, 242.

Fierz, W., Brenan, M., Müllbacher, A. & Simpson, E. (1982a) Non H-2 and H-2 linked immune response genes control the cytotoxic T-cell response to H-Y. *Immunogenetics*, **15**, 261.

Fierz, W., Farmer, G. A., Sheena, J. H. & Simpson, E. (1982b) Genetic analysis of the non H-2 linked Ir genes controlling the cytotoxic T cell response to H-Y in H-2^d mice. *Immunogenetics*, **16**, 593.

Fujiwara, H. & Shearer, G. M. (1981) Non H-2 associated genetic regulation of cytotoxic responses to hapten-modified syngeneic cells. Effect on the magnitude of secondary response and helper T cell generation after *in vivo* priming. *Eur. J. Immunol.* **11**, 700.

Gascoigne, N. R. J. (1983) The regulation of the immune response to minor alloantigens. *PhD Thesis*, London University.

Gasser, D. L. & Silvers, W. K. (1972) Genetics and immunology of sex-linked antigens. *Adv. Immunol.* **15**, 215.

Gasser, D. L., Silvers, W. K. & Wachtel, S. S. (1974) Sex-associated antigens in mice and rats. *Science*, **185**, 963.

Goldberg, E. H., Boyse, E. A., Scheid, M. & Bennett, D. (1972) Production of H-Y antibodies by female mice that fail to reject male skin. *Nature (Lond.)*, **238**, 55.

Gordon, R. D., Samelson, L. & Simpson, E. (1975) *In vitro* cell-mediated immune responses to the male specific (H-Y) antigen in mice. *J. exp. Med.* **142**, 1349.

Gordon, R. D., Samelson, L. & Simpson, E. (1977) Selective response to H-Y antigen by F_1 female mice sensitized to F_1 male cells. *J. exp. Med.* **146**, 606.

Gordon, R. D. & Simpson, E. (1977) Immune response gene control of cytotoxic T cell responses to H-Y. *Transplant. Proc.* **9**, 885.

Gordon, R. D., Simpson, E. & Samelson, L. E. (1975) *In vitro* cell mediated immune responses to the male specific (H-Y) antigen in mice. *J. exp. Med.* **142**, 1108.

Greene, M. I., Benacerraf, B. & Dorf, M. E. (1980) The characterisation of the delayed-type hypersensitivity reaction to H-Y antigens. *Immunogenetics*, **11**, 267.

Hauschka, T. S. (1955) Probable Y linkage of a histocompatibility gene. *Transplant. Bull.* **2**, 154.

Hurme, M., Chandler, P. R., Hetherington, C. M. & Simpson, E. (1978b) Cytotoxic T-cell responses to H-Y: correlation with the rejection of syngeneic male skin grafts. *J. exp. Med.* **147**, 768.

Hurme, M., Hetherington, C. H., Chandler, P. R., Gordon, R. D. & Simpson, E. (1977) Cytotoxic T-cell responses to H-Y: Ir genes and associative antigens map in H-2. *Immunogenetics*, **5**, 453.

Hurme, M., Hetherington, C. M., Chandler, P. R. & Simpson, E. (1978a) Cytotoxic T cell responses to H-Y: mapping of the Ir genes. *J. exp. Med.* **147**, 758.

Johnson, L. L. (1982) A protocol for detection of H-Y antigenic variants. *Immunogenetics*, **16**, 577.

Johnson, L. L., Bailey, D. W. & Mobraaten, L. E. (1981) Genetics of histocompatibility in mice. IV. Detection of certain minor (non H-2) H antigens in selected organs by the popliteal lymph node test. *Immunogenetics*, **14**, 63.

Johnson, L. L., Sargent, E. C., Washburn, L. L. & Eicher, E. M. (1983) XY Female mice express H-Y antigens. *Devel. Genet.* **3**, 247.

Klein, J. (1975) *Biology of the Mouse Histocompatibility-2 Complex*. Springer Verlag, New York.

Liew, F. Y. & Simpson, E. (1980) Delayed-type hypersensitivity responses to H-Y: characterization and mapping of Ir genes. *Immunogenetics*, **11**, 255.

McLaren, A. & Monk, M. (1982) Fertile females produced by inactivation of an X-chromosome of 'sex reversed' mice. *Nature (Lond.)*, **300**, 446.

McClaren, A., Simpson, E., Tomonari, K., Chandler, P. & Hogg, H. (1984) Male sexual differentiation in mice lacking H-Y antigen. *Nature (Lond.)* (in press).

Melvold, R. W., Koln, H. I., Yerganian, G. & Fawcett, D. W. (1977) Evidence suggesting the existence of two H-Y antigens in the mouse. *Immunogenetics*, **5**, 33.

Michaelides, M., Sandrin, M. S., Morgan, G., McKenzie, I. F. C., Ashman, R. & Melvold, R. W. (1981) Ir gene function in an I-A subregion mutant B6.C-H-2 bm12. *J. exp. Med.* **153**, 464.

Mintz, B. & Silvers, W. K. (1983) Graft evidence for H-Y transplantation antigen similarity in different mouse strains. *Immunogenetics*, **17**, 533.

Müllbacher, A., Sheena, J. H., Fierz, W. & Brenan, M. (1981) Specific haplotype preference in congenic F_1 hybrid mice in the cytotoxic T cell response to the male specific antigen H-Y. *J. Immunol.* **127**, 686.

Ohno, S. (1977) The original function of MHC antigens as the general plasma membrane anchorage site for organogenesis-directing proteins. *Immunol. Rev.* **33**, 59.

Pole, D. & Simpson, E. (1983) Genetic control and effector cells in host versus graft responses to H-Y antigen in mice. *Transplantation* (in press).

Shearer, G. M. (1974) Cell mediated cytotoxicity to TNP modified syngeneic lymphocytes. *Eur. J. Immunol.* **4**, 527.

Silvers, W. K., Gasser, D. L. & Eicher, E. M. (1982) The H-Y antigen, serologically detectable male antigens and sex determination. *Cell*, **28**, 439.

Simon, M. M., Edwards, A. J., Hammerling, U., McKenzie, I. F. C., Eichmann, K. & Simpson, E. (1981). Generation of effector cells for T cell subsets. III. Synergy between Lyt-1 and Lyt-123/23 lymphocytes in the generation of H-2 restricted and alloreactive cytotoxic T cells. *Eur. J. Immun.* **11**, 246.

Simpson, E. (1982) The role of H-Y as a minor transplantation antigen. *Immunol. Today*, **3**, 97.

Simpson, E., Benjamin, D. & Chandler, P. (1981a) Non-responsiveness to H-Y: tolerance in H-2^b mice. *Transplant. Proc.* **13**, 1880.

Simpson, E., Brunner, C., Hetherinton, C., Chandler, P., Brenan, M., Dagg, M. & Bailey, D. W. (1979) H-Y antigen: no evidence for alleles in wild strains of mice. *Immunogenetics*, **8**, 213.

Simpson, E., Chandler, P., Liew, F. Y., Farmer, G., Fierz, W. & Gregory, R. (1983a) Induction and effector function of T cells. In: *Genetics of the Immune Response* (eds G. and E. Moller), p. 121. Plenum Press.

Simpson, E., Chandler, P., Washburn, L. L., Bunker, H. P. & Eicher, E. M. (1983b) H-Y typing of karyotypically abnormal mice. *Differentiation*, **23** (Suppl.), S116.

Simpson, E., Edwards, P., Wachtel, S., McLaren, A. & Chandler, P. (1981b). H-Y antigen in Sxr mice detected by H-2 restricted cytotoxic T cells. *Immunogenetics*, **13**, 355.

Simpson, E. & Gordon, R. D. (1977) Responsiveness to H-Y antigen: Ir gene complementation and target cell specificity. *Immunol. Rev.* **35**, 59.

Simpson, E., McLaren, A. & Chandler, P. (1982) Evidence for two male antigens in mice. *Immunogenetics*, **15**, 609.

Simpson, E., McLaren, A., Chandler, P. & Tomonari, K. (1984) Expression of H-Y antigen by female mice carrying *Sxr*. *Transplantation*, **127** (in press).

Snell, G. D. (1956) A comment on Eichwald & Silmser's communication. *Transplant. Bull.* **3**, 29.

Tomonari, K. (1983a) Antigen and MHC restriction specificity of two types of cloned male specific T cell lines. *J. Immunol.* **131**, 1641.

Tomonari, K. (1983b) *In vitro* and *in vivo* helper activity of an H-Y specific, IA^b restricted T cell clone for the H-Y specific cytotoxic T lymphocyte response. (Submitted).

von Boehmer, H., Hengartner, H., Nabholz, M., Lernhardt, W., Schreier, M. H. &

Haas, W. (1979) Fine specificity of a continuously growing iller cell clone specific for H-Y antigen. *Eur. J. Immunol.* **9**, 592.

Wachtel, S. S., Ohno, O., Koo, G. C. & Boyse, E. A. (1975) Possible role for H-Y antigen in the primary determination of sex. *Nature (Lond.)*, **257**, 235.

Wettstein, P. J. & Frelinger, J. A. (1980) H-2 effects on cell–cell interactions in the response to single non H-2 alloantigens. III. Evidence for a second Ir-gene system mapping in the H-2K and H-2D regions. *Immunogenetics*, **10**, 211.

Zinkernagel, R. M. & Doherty, P. C. (1974) Restriction of *in vitro* T cell mediated cytotoxicity in LCM within a syngeneic or semiallogeneic system. *Nature (Lond.)*, **248**, 701.

Chapter 6
Molecular genetics of the HLA-D region

W. Bodmer, Julia Bodmer, Janet Lee, A. So, R. Spielman,
P. Travers & J. Trowsdale

Imperial Cancer Research Fund, Lincoln's Inn Fields, London WC2A 3PX

Summary. The HLA-D region or class II antigens have been shown to consist of three major sets of products: DR, DC and SB.* Each product consists of non-covalently associated polypeptide chains α and β each of which has two protein domains outside the cell, followed by a transmembrane region and a short intracytoplasmic tail. Cloning the HLA-D region products has shown that there are at least six α chain genes and probably seven or more β chain genes, and that in most and probably all cases, α and β chains for a given set of products occur together in clusters within the HLA-D region. Of the α chains, only DCα shows extensive polymorphism, while much of the serologically detected polymorphism is associated with β chains, especially those of the DR and DC antigens. The variation is most easily understood in terms of natural selection acting to generate polymorphism because of differences in immune response. Sequence and structural comparisons between HLA-D region and other HLA products, as well as immunoglobulins, show them to be members of a larger family of related proteins, with functions defined mainly within the immune system and involving predominantly cellular interactions.

Introduction

The HLA-D region or class II antigens were first defined by cellular methods using the mixed lymphocyte culture test (MLC). The initial antigens defined by MLC were assigned to the HLA-D locus as a series of alleles expressed on B lymphocytes (Kissmeyer-Nielsen, 1975). Shortly afterwards, serological approaches to the definition of class II antigens on B lymphocytes were developed, paralleling those which led to the definition of the HLA-ABC products (Bodmer *et al.*, 1978; Bodmer, 1978), and the corresponding antigens were called HLA-DR for D-related

---

* Since this paper was written, the WHO Nomenclature Committee for HLA have renamed two of the HLA-D subregions. DQ is what was formerly DC, and DP is the new name for SB. DR remains unchanged.

antigens. Subsequently, two further sets of antigens, called DC and SB, were defined by a combination of serological, cellular and biochemical techniques. The DC (also sometimes called MT or MB) products were originally defined by cross-reacting groups of DR antigens, including especially DR1, 2 and w6. Tosi *et al.* (1978) suggested that these patterns corresponded to the products of a second locus in addition to DR, which they called DC, whose alleles were in strong linkage disequilibrium with those at the DR locus, accounting for the established patterns of apparent cross-reactions. The confirmation of the DC locus and its products came through the use of monoclonal antibodies for immunochemical analysis, in particular using immunoprecipitation followed by two-dimensional gel analysis to distinguish the DC from the DR products (for review see Shackelford *et al.*, 1982; Bodmer & Bodmer, 1984). The SB locus was defined by cellular methods, using the primed lymphocyte typing approach, by Shaw *et al.* (1981). In this case also, putative identification of the products came from the use of monoclonal antibodies (Shackelford *et al.*, 1982; Bodmer & Bodmer, 1984).

Following the initial serological definition of the HLA-DR antigens it was shown that these were composed of two non-covalently associated glycosylated transmembrane polypeptides of molecular weights 33,000 (α) and 28,000 (β). In the mouse H-2 immune response or I region, a homologous set of antigens has been defined, called I-A and I-E, which have the same structure. Amino acid sequence comparisons between the corresponding human and mouse products show clearly that I-A corresponds to DC, while I-E corresponds to DR. A schematic comparison of the genetic maps of the H-2 and HLA regions, showing the correspondence between the H-2 I and HLA-D regions, is shown in Fig. 6.1. The alignment maximizes the homology between the two regions, placing the complement components coded for in the major histocompatibility regions between the class I (H-2 DL and HLA-ABC) and the class II H-2 I and HLA-D genes. Only the class I H-2 K locus is left out of line on the centromeric side of the H-2 I region. The sequence of the HLA-SB, DC and DR sets of genes as shown in Fig. 6.1 fits in with the known H-2 I region sequence of the I-A and I-E genes, and agrees with the data obtained using deletion mutants (De Mars *et al.*, 1983).

A third polypeptide chain, called the invariant I chain, was first identified in the mouse by Jones, Murphy & McDevitt (1978) as a chain associated with the H-2 I region α and β chains, at least inside the cell. This chain was later identified in man by Charron & McDevitt (1979) and others, and was shown by Owen *et al.* (1981) to be associated almost exclusively with the α and β chain inside the cell, and not on the cell surface. The invariant I chain is extensively glycosylated and shows a number of processing variants, depending on the addition of various sugar side chains and sialic residues (Rudd *et al.*, 1984). The genes for this chain have been cloned (Long *et al.*, 1983; Claesson *et al.*, 1983) and have been shown not to map to chromosome 6. Though they are clearly important for the function of the HLA-D region products, they will not be discussed further in this paper.

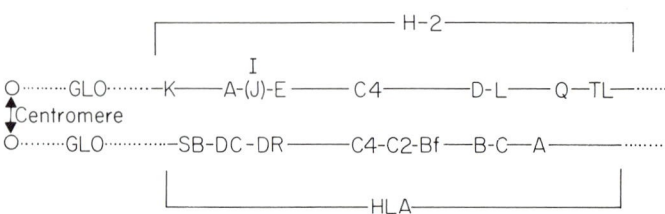

Fig. 6.1. Schematic comparison of genetic maps of the mouse H-2 and human HLA regions. GLO is the linked marker enzyme glyoxylase. H-2 is on mouse chromosome 17 and HLA on the short arm of human chromosome 6. K, D, L are the classical H-2 class I transplantation antigens, whose human equivalents are A, B and C. Q and TL are related class I products which are differentiation antigens on certain types of lymphocytes. C4, C2 and BF are, respectively, the fourth and second classical complement components and factor B of the alternate pathway, whose genes lie in the H-2 and HLA regions. The H-2 I region in the mouse was initially defined through the control of immune response. Subsequently antigens, mainly present on B lymphocytes, were separately defined in the I-A and I-E regions. In humans the equivalent of the I region is the D region which includes the genes for at least three sets of products, SB, DR and DC. Each of these is coded for by sets of α and β chain genes. DR corresponds to mouse I-E, and DC to mouse I-A, while SB has no mouse equivalent. The genetic maps in mouse and man are aligned to give maximum homology between the species.

Protein and nucleic acid sequence data have indicated that the HLA-D region α and β chains each have two protein domains outside the cell, followed by a transmembrane region and a short intracytoplasmic tail. The HLA class I or ABC products, in contrast, have three external protein domains, but the product with which they associate, namely β_2m, has only a single domain which is thought to associate with the HLA-ABC product domain closest to the membrane. Thus both sets of products can be drawn with a similar schematic structure, as shown in Fig. 6.2. The aim of this paper is to give a brief review, emphasizing our own studies, of the molecular analysis of the HLA-D region products. This has provided information concerning the number of genes in the region, the structural and evolutionary relationships amongst these genes, and between them and the HLA-ABC and other products, and the patterns of variations of the HLA-D region products and their functional significance.

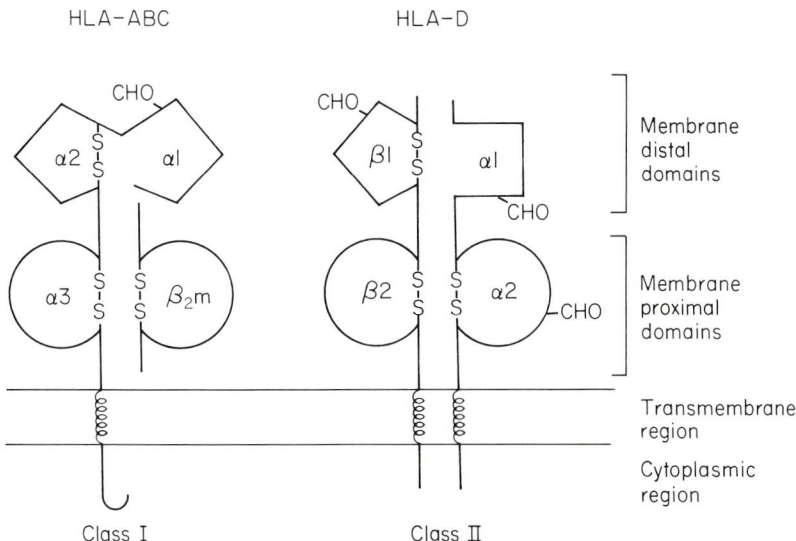

Fig. 6.2. Schematic structure of HLA class I and class II glycoproteins. The membrane proximal and membrane distal domains are shown aligned according to the predicted analogy with immunoglobulin structure. The positions of internal disulphide bridges (S-S) and carbohydrate side chains (CHO) are indicated. The similarity of shapes of the membrane proximal domains, and of the membrane distal domains ABC $\alpha1$, $\alpha2$ and HLA-D $\beta1$ indicates that they form two classes of related sequences within the overall class of immunoglobulin related structures. (From Bodmer *et al.*, 1984.)

Cloning the HLA-D region

Initially cDNA clones for the HLA-DR α and certain other chains were obtained using a variety of approaches by several laboratories (for a review, see Trowsdale *et al.*, 1984a). These clones were then used to obtain genomic clones for the analysis of the organization of the individual genes for the different chains, with a view to establishing the overall structure of the HLA-D region at the molecular level. In our laboratory, a cDNA clone for the HLA-DR α chain was isolated (Lee, Trowsdale & Bodmer, 1982a), and comparison of the sequences of this clone with a genomic clone containing the corresponding gene revealed its intron–exon structure (Lee *et al.*, 1982b). The translated sequence of the cDNA clone suggested an extra-cellular two domain organization of the corresponding protein, with the domain nearest the membrane having a disulphide bridge characteristic of immunoglobulin domains. Similar data were obtained for a cDNA clone for a β chain gene by Larhammar *et al.* (1982). These and other sequence data (for a review, see e.g. Shackelford *et al.*, 1982; Steinmetz & Hood, 1983) have shown that the membrane proximal domains of the α and β chains of the HLA-D region, the corresponding domains of the HLA-ABC products, β_2m and the immunoglobulin constant regions form a family of closely related structures, as will be discussed further below. The other major feature to come from these analyses is that the structure of the genes at the genomic level reveals a striking correspondence between presumptive protein domains and exons, as has been found for other major histocompatibility system products as well as for the immunoglobulins and other genes. A schematic diagram comparing the genomic organization of HLA-ABC, and HLA-D region α and β chains is shown in Fig. 6.3. The class II β chain genes have an extra intron in their transmembrane and cytoplasmic region, making them somewhat more analogous to the class I than to the class II α chains in this particular respect.

Using the HLA-DR α cDNA clone, a number of cosmids containing related sequences have been isolated in our laboratory (Trowsdale *et al.*, 1983). One of these cosmids contained the sequence corresponding to the cDNA clone for the DR α chain itself, and formed the basis for analysing

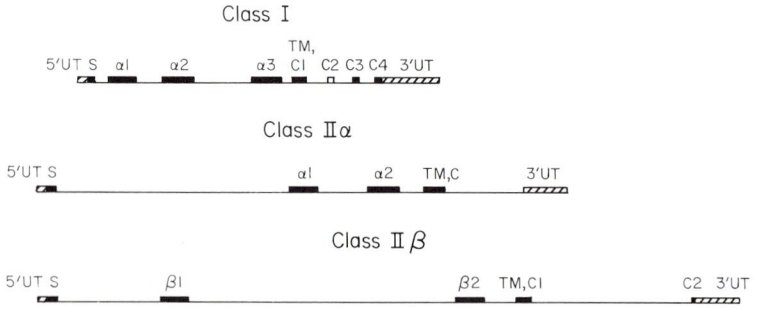

Fig. 6.3. Schematic diagrams comparing the genomic organizations of class I, class II α and class II β chain genes. 5′UT = 5′ untranslated; 3′UT = 3′ untranslated. α1, α2, α3, β1, β2 = protein domains; TM = transmembrane; C, C1, etc. = cytoplasmic sequences. Relative lengths are approximate. See text for appropriate references.

its genomic structure. Another pair of overlapping cosmids contained a different α chain which, on the basis of sequence analysis, was shown clearly to correspond to a DC α chain. A further pair of cosmids, which overlap considerably, were shown to contain yet another α chain gene different from both DR and DC, which was suggested to be an SB α chain (Trowsdale *et al.*, 1983), a suggestion that has subsequently been confirmed by sequence analysis (unpublished data). Using human–mouse somatic cell hybrids which segregate for chromosome 6, the chromosome containing the HLA region, it has been clearly shown that these α chains all map to chromosome 6, and so are presumably in the HLA region (Lee *et al.*, 1982a; Trowsdale *et al.*, 1983).

Three further α chains have been identified, in addition to those already described corresponding to DR α, DC α and SB α. The first of these was identified by Southern blot analysis, using a DC α-specific probe, which showed the existence of a second closely related gene, that has been called DX α. The second of the new α chain genes is a further sequence identified on the overlapping cosmids containing the originally identified SB α indicating that, as for DC, there are two closely related SB α genes which we have called SB α1 and SB α2 (Spielman *et al.*, 1984). Lastly, a further cosmid has been identified containing a complete α chain gene that appears to be different from any of the others, though obviously related to them in sequence. All of these six α chain genes appear to map to the HLA region, but it is not yet known how many of them are expressed, though at least three must be, corresponding respectively to DR, DC and SB.

A combination of a search for sequences on these cosmids that are expressed in B cells, other than those corresponding to the α chain genes, and the use of an HLA-DC β cDNA clone kindly given to us by Drs Larhammar and Peterson, has shown that at least three of the cosmids which contain α chain genes also carry β chain genes (Lee *et al.*, 1983; Bodmer *et al.*, 1984). Thus the SB α-carrying cosmids have a β gene between the two α genes, and another cosmid has at least one β chain gene to the 3' side of the DC α gene. Sequence analysis indicates that the β chain sequences correspond to their neighbouring α chain sequences, and thus that α and β chains for the DC and SB sets of products occur together. For the SB subregion, a more detailed analysis has shown that there is a pair of α and β genes occurring in the sequence SB α1, SB β1, SB α2, SB β2, suggesting that the original SB αβ pair were duplicated, perhaps comparatively recently in evolution (Trowsdale *et al.*, 1984). Southern blot analysis (Wake, Long & Mach, 1982; Bodmer *et al.*, 1984), using β chain sequence probes suggests that there may be as many as 10–15 β chain genes, though once again how many of these are expressed is not yet clear.

D region polymorphism at the DNA level

Restriction enzyme polymorphisms, detected using cloned DNA probes from the HLA region, provide a major new source of genetic variants that can be used to analyse in greater depth the serological and functional variation controlled by the HLA region, including in particular its association with disease, and matching for transplantation. Analysis of the protein products of the HLA-D region, mainly using immunochemical techniques, has indicated that the major polymorphism is with respect to the β chains, though limited variation for the DC α chain on two-dimensional gels has been described (De Kretser *et al.*, 1982; for a review of this, see Bodmer & Bodmer, 1984). The first results obtained by Wake *et al.* (1982) and Bodmer *et al.* (1984) using β chain probes for the detection of restriction enzyme polymorphisms clearly indicated a high degree of variation associated with at least some of these genes. By contrast, and perhaps as expected, no polymorphism was initially seen using the DR α chain probe (Lee *et al.*, 1982a). However, when a DC α probe was used extensive polymorphism was revealed, which segregated as expected in at least one family. More particularly this variation correlated, when using the restriction enzyme EcoR1, with the serological patterns of DR cross-reaction that formed the initial basis of the definition of the DC variants (Trowsdale *et al.*, 1983; Auffray *et al.*, 1983). At the same time it was shown that the DX α gene, closely related to DC α, showed limited variation, but perhaps more than that seen for DR α and SB α. Further analysis has confirmed and extended these results. Thus Spielman *et al.* (1984) have shown that of the six α chain genes so far identified, only DC α shows extensive polymorphism with a variety of restriction enzymes, DX α shows limited polymorphism, while the remaining α genes are substantially less polymorphic than either of these two and show variation only exceptionally. A summary of the properties of the six different α chains defined so far is shown in Table 6.1.

The patterns of variation on Southern blots and their association with serological types are established using, for the most part, Epstein–Barr virus-transformed lymphoblastoid cell lines from HLA homozygotes. In those cases where the individuals from whom the lines were grown out are known to be homozygous because they come from consanguineous

Table 6.1. Summary of characterization of HLA-DR α related genes on chromosome 6

Gene	Characteristic band sizes in kb (approx.)		
	EcoR1	Pst1	
DR	3·2, 4·5	2·0, 5·8	
DZ	10·0	2·0	
DC	variable (15·5)	variable (12·5)	closely related
DX	5·0	variable (6·6)	
SB1	11·0	1·9, 2·3	closely linked
SB2	5·5	3·2	

Except in the case of the DC α and DX α genes, the band sizes obtained on Southern blots of human genomic DNA are identical to those present in cosmid clones. Because of the polymorphism of these two genes, characteristic sizes for a DRw6 cell line are shown. All of the band sizes are approximate, and those above 10 kb may not be very accurate.

(From Spielman *et al.*, 1984).

parents, the homozygosity is more securely established. These lines are very convenient tools for analysing the variation, since its pattern is simpler in homozygotes than heterozygotes and, in addition, in homozygotes variations due to polymorphism can more easily be distinguished from those due to differences between loci. A summary of data obtained using a DC α chain probe for analysis of restriction enzyme digests of DNA from a series of such cell lines with EcoR1 and Taq1, is shown in Table 6.2. The patterns detected using EcoR1 correspond very clearly with the HLA-DR cross-reactive serotypes (DR1, 2, w6; DR3, 5; DR4, 7) that are associated with variation at the DC or MT locus. This includes, for example, the classification of Koz, a DRw9 cell, with MT3, and of FPF with MT1, this being a DR5 homozygote cell line that unusually has the MT1 serological type. The pattern revealed for DC sequences by Taq1 digestion appears to associate as much with the DR as with the MT classification, suggesting that different parts of the DC sequence are revealing their polymorphism using these two enzymes. The DX gene shows limited variation only with the enzymes Taq1 and Pst1. Some

Table 6.2. The correspondence between HLA-DR types and restriction enzyme fragment haplotypes detected by the DC α chain probe

Cell		HLA-ABC	DR	MT	EcoR1		TaQ1	
					DC	DX	DC	DX
Maja		A2; Bw35; Cw4	1	1	15·5*	5·0	2·6	1·9/2·1
Mette		A2, 3; B5, 18; NT	1	1	15·5	5·0	2·6	a‡
Hom2		A3; B27; C1	1	1	15·5	5·0	2·6	a
IBW4	C†	A3; B27; C1	1	1	15·5	5·0	2·6	a
MST		A3; B7; NT	2	1	15·5	5·0	5·3	2·1
PGF	C	A3; B7; NT	2	1	15·5	5·0	5·3	a
WT18	C	A2; B27; Cw2	2	1	15·5	5·0	5·3	a
BBF	C	A1; B37; Cw6	2	1	15·5	5·0	5·3	a
Daudi			w6	1	15·5	5·0	6·4	a
WVB	C	A2; B16; NT	w6	1	15·5	5·0	6·4	a
WT46	C	A32; B13; NT	w6	1	15·5	5·0	5·3	a
WT52	C	A11; B22; Cw3	w6	1	15·5	5·0	2·6	a
Arnt		A2; Bw38; w39; NT	w6	1	15·5	5·0	6·4	a
FpF	C	A1; Bw35; Cw4	5	1	15·5	5·0	6·4	a

WT49	C	A2; B17; NT	3	2	12·3	5·0	4·3	1·9
WT20	C	A30; B18; Cw5	3	2	12·5	5·0	4·3	a
SCTA		A1; B8; Cw4	3	2	12·5	5·0	4·3	a
Herluf		A2; B12; w35; Cw4, 5	H	2	12·5	5·0	4·3	a
IDF		A26, 2/28; Bw38, 18; NT	5	2	12·5	5·0	4·3	1·9
1296-S		A2; Bw51, 44; NT	4	3	6·2	5·0	4·8	1·9/2·1
JHH		A2; B15; Cw3	4	3	6·2	5·0	4·7	2·1
WT51	C	A9; B14; NT	4	3	6·2	5·0	NT	a
Mann	C	A29; B12; Cw4	7	3	6·2	5·0	4·8	1·9
IBW9	C	Aw33; B14; Cw8	7	3	6·2	5·0	4·8	2·1
TF6		A1; B17; NT	7	3	6·2	5·0	4·8	a
Koz		Aw24, 26; Bw54, 40; NT	w9	3	6·2	5·0	4·8	1·9
Priess		A2; B15; Cw3	4	3	15·5/12·5	5·0	4·3/2·6	2·1

* Approximate sizes (in kb) of polymorphic fragments are averages from five (EcoR1) or three (Taq1) gels. The gels do not permit a very accurate measure of the sizes of the bands, particularly those over 10·0 kb.

† C, from consanguineous parents.

‡ a, 2·0 kb band(s) were present, but gels to resolve 1·9 and 2·0 kb bands were not run.

NT, not tested.

Some of the MT (DC) types are inferred: not all of the lines have been typed for MT.

(From Spielman *et al.*, 1984.)

evidence has also been obtained for variation in the number of genes as well as in their restriction enzyme sites, in some of the homozygous typing on lines (A. So, unpublished data).

As already mentioned, extensive polymorphism is revealed using β chain probes. It appears that the β chains have more sequences in common between them so that, for example, an SB β probe picks up DC and DR β variations. To obtain a more refined analysis of the variation for individual DC β, DR β and SB β genes, it is necessary to use subclones for distinctive parts of the genes, such as their intron sequences or 3' untranslated regions of the mRNAs from cDNA clones. In this case it can be shown that certain patterns correlate clearly with the DR serology, others with the DC serology, while the known SB β gene associates with the SB based cellular typing (A. So, personal communication). Preliminary data suggest that the SB β genes are less variable than the others, but more work is needed to sort out the pattern of variation for this complex set of genes.

The high level of variation found at the DNA level with the DC α probe, in contrast to the relative lack of variation for the other α chain genes, matches the relatively high level of variation found in the mouse for the homologous I-A α chain genes by Benoist *et al.* (1983) and Chang, Moriuchi & Silver (1983). These authors have also shown that the polymorphic variation is associated, as expected, predominantly with the N terminal membrane distal domain and, more particularly, with particular regions of this domain such as between amino acids 10 and 15, 56 to 57 and around 75 to 80. Similar data have also been obtained for the β chain variation (see e.g. Larhammar *et al.*, 1983). The striking contrast in the level of variation for the DC α chain as compared to the other α chains can only satisfactorily be explained by natural selection acting on DC α polymorphic variants. This suggests that this product has greater functional significance for the generation of immune response differences (and consequent resistance to viral, bacterial or protozoan parasites) than have the other α chain genes. As often discussed before (see e.g. Bodmer, 1972), the serologically detected polymorphism is most easily understood in terms of natural selection acting to generate polymorphism because of variations in immune response. Presumably the variable regions within the membrane distal domains are those parts of the molecule which play a functional role in immune response differences, and so where variation in amino acid sequence can more readily lead to the generation of differences in immune response. These results strongly suggest, therefore, that some of the HLA-D region disease associations may involve DC α

chain variations, as well as variations for the various β chains which were previously thought to be the major source of polymorphism in the region. As has been suggested by Bodmer *et al.* (1984) and Spielman *et al.* (1984), the association of insulin-dependent juvenile onset diabetes mellitus with both DR3 and DR4 might most easily, in the light of these data, be explained by an association with a particular DC $\alpha\beta$ chain combination determinant.

Structure and evolution of HLA-D region products

The membrane proximal domains of the sets of class I and class II HLA region products, whose overall structure is indicated schematically in Fig. 6.2, show, as already mentioned, the greatest similarity to each other and with immunoglobulin constant region domains. The amino acid sequences of these domains can be aligned by the position of the cysteines which form the basis for disulphide bridges, and by certain other highly conserved residues found, in particular, in the neighbourhood of the cysteines. Using such an alignment, the overall similarity between the various domains is between 20 and 30%, as measured by the percentage of amino acids in common between pairs of sequences. Data for a set of sequences of D region α and β chains, as well as class I products, β_2m and a human immunoglobulin constant region of a λ light chain are summarized in Table 6.3. These data clearly show the homology between DR and I-E, and DC and I-A, and also show that DR and DC differ from each other by about as much as the species differences between homologous human and mouse products. Alpha and β chains, on the other hand, differ from each other very substantially, almost as much as do the class I and class II products from each other, or either of them from β_2m or immunoglobulin constant regions. The pattern of divergence clearly suggests that the HLA region consists of a set of genes with a common origin by duplication from an ancestral gene. The most recent separation is presumably that between the two sets of SB products mentioned above, (and possibly between DC and DX) followed by the differences between DR, DC and SB. Next, going back in time, are presumably the differences between α and β chains, then between class I and class II products, and finally between HLA region products overall and immunoglobulins and β_2m. The whole of this latter set of divergences, including that between α and β chain genes happened, perhaps, between 500 and 700 million years ago. Indeed, since the differences between α and β chains are not much less than those between HLA region

Table 6.3. Homologies between membrane proximal domains of MHC-related proteins and immunoglobulin constant domains

	DR-α2	I-Eα2	DC-α2	I-Aα2	DR-β2	DC-β2	ABC	ψABC	H-2	β₂m	Cλ
DR-α2	—	88	62	58	32	32	28	29	21	26	26
I-Eα2		—	66	61	30	31	26	28	20	28	27
DC-α2			—	72	28	27	25	25	19	26	27
I-Aα2				—	28	28	24	25	18	27	23
DR-β2					—	68	28	28	27	31	31
DC-β2						—	29	29	25	27	28
ABC							—	94	68	21	22
ψABCα3								—	69	20	20
H-2Kᵇα3									—	20	17
β₂m										—	16
Cλ											—

The number of identical residues between each pair of sequences is shown. The total length of sequence compared is 98 amino acids, so these figures approximate to the percentage homology between the sequences compared. For details concerning the sequences used, see Travers *et al.* (1984).

products and immunoglobulins, the data suggest a relatively rapid evolution of these various products, starting between 600 and 800 million years ago at about the time of the major initial divergence of the vertebrates. This time probably corresponded to the period when there was greatest pressure for the initial evolution of the immune system, and so on its diversification (Bodmer *et al.*, 1984; Travers *et al.*, 1984).

Alignment of the various membrane proximal domain sequences reveals a number of conserved residues characteristic of the immunoglobulin β pleated sheet structure. Using the known crystal structure of an immunoglobulin fragment and computer graphic techniques, it has been possible to obtain a detailed structure prediction for the DR α and β chain membrane proximal domain combination (Travers *et al.*, 1984). The model provides a consistent explanation for conserved residues which are predicted to be involved in maintaining the β barrel structure and the interactions between α and β chain domains. The need for such specific interaction, and the pattern of amino acid sequence divergence between the different sets of products, readily explains, and indeed predicts, the lack of association between α chains from one locus and β chains from another. The model also provides an intriguing explanation for the unusual degree of homology of the transmembrane sequences of different HLA-D region α and different β chains. The α and β chains are suggested to pack together tightly within the membrane.

The similarities between the membrane distal domains and immunoglobulin regions are too low to allow for specific structure predictions analogous to those made for the membrane proximal domains. Their sequences, however, suggest that they might also fold to form a β barrel structure, and it is tempting to suggest that their topology may be more similar to that of immunoglobulin-variable than constant region domains.

Conclusions

The HLA-D region or class II products are clearly members of a larger family of related proteins with functions so far defined mainly within the immune system, and involving predominantly cellular interactions. This family includes the class I and class II HLA region products, the immunoglobulins, β_2m and the T cell differentiation antigen Thy-1 (see e.g. Lee *et al.*, 1982b; Williams & Gagnon, 1982). It is intriguing that the suggestion that HLA region and immunoglobulin products might be related and involve both ligands and receptors for molecules involved in cellular interactions (Bodmer, 1972) is supported by this body of molecular data, as well as by the recent demonstration that immunoglobulin receptors (Mostov, Friedlander & Blobel, 1984) and the T lymphocyte receptor (Hedrik *et al.*, 1984) are members of this same family. The mouse H-2 region appears to contain mainly the I-A, and the I-E α and β chain genes (Steinmetz & Hood, 1983). Thus the human HLA-D region is clearly much more complex since, apart from containing the third class of products SB not so far identified in the mouse, it also contains a wider variety of the DR, I-E and DC, I-A related sets of genes. From the extent of sequence divergence between SB and DR or DC, it seems likely that these genes arose relatively early during mammalian evolution, and so that rodents have lost all or most of the SB gene sequences during their evolution. As discussed by Trowsdale *et al.* (1984) and Bodmer (1984), a possible reason for the greater complexity of the human HLA-D region may lie in the fact that this complexity is an advantage to the longer-lived species, in giving it a greater opportunity for producing rapid and flexible variations in immune response to cope with novel pathogens.

Clearly the major challenge for further work on the HLA-D region, and of course its class I counterparts, is to complete the structural analysis with a view to relating structure and function, and in particular to achieving a detailed understanding of the role of the HLA system in immune response, disease susceptibility and transplantation matching. Intriguing questions remain to be answered concerning the tissue distribution of HLA-D region products, which is mainly on B lymphocytes, macrophages and dendritic cells, but also sometimes on endothelial cells, some epithelial cells and melanocytes. Molecular probes will play an important part in analysing this tissue distribution and the conditions under which HLA-D region products may be expressed, particularly following certain types of immune stimuli (for a review, see Bodmer & Bodmer, 1984). As already emphasized, analysis of variation at the DNA level using restriction enzymes and Southern blotting is revealing new variations that may be of considerable significance for understanding immune response differences and disease susceptibility. The challenge here is clearly to identify the specific sequence differences that determine variations in immune response. All of these structural and functional analyses will be greatly aided by a complete genomic map of the HLA-D region and an analysis of its expressed products.

References

Auffray, C., Ben-Nun, A., Roux-Dosseto, M., Germain, R. N., Seidman, J. G. & Strominger, J. L. (1983) Polymorphism and complexity of the human DC and murine I-A α-chain genes. *EMBO J.* **2(1)**, 121.

Benoist, B. O., Mathis, D. J., Kanter, M. R., Williams, V. E. II & McDevitt, H. O. (1983) Regions of allelic hypervariability in the murine A_α immune response gene. *Cell*, **34**, 169.

Bodmer, J. G. (1978) Ia antigens: definition of the HLA-DRW specificities. *Br. med. Bull.* **34(3)**, 233.

Bodmer, J. G. & Bodmer, W. F. (1984) Monoclonal antibodies to HLA determinants. *Br. med. Bull.* **40(3)**, 267.

Bodmer, W. F. (1972) Evolutionary significance of the HL-A system. *Nature (Lond.)*, **237**, 139.

Bodmer, W. F. (1984) The major histocompatibility system: structure and function: summary and synthesis. In: *Proceedings of the Fifth International Immunology Congress, Kyoto, Japan*, p. 959. Academic Press.

Bodmer, W. F., Batchelor, J. R., Bodmer, J. G., Festenstein, H. & Morris, P. J., eds (1978) *Histocompatibility Testing 1977. Report of the Seventh International Histocompatibility Workshop and Conference.* Munksgaard, Copenhagen.

Bodmer, W., Bodmer, J., Lee, J., Spielman, R., Travers, P. & Trowsdale, J. (1984) Structure, Evolution and Polymorphism of the HLA-D Region. *Tokyo Symposium on Immunogenetics—its Applications to Clinical Medicine* (in press). Japan Medical Research Foundation.

Chang, H. C., Moriuchi, T. & Silver, J. (1983) The heavy chain of human B-cell alloantigen HLA-DS has a variable N-terminal region and a constant immunoglobulin-like region. *Nature (Lond.)*, **305**, 813.

Charron, D. J. & McDevitt, H. O. (1979) Analysis of HLA-D region-associated molecules with monoclonal antibody. *Proc. natn. Acad. Sci. U.S.A.* **76**, 6567.

Claesson, L., Larhammar, D., Rask, L. & Peterson, P. A. (1983) cDNA clone for the human invariant γ-chain of Class II histocompatibility antigens and its implications for the protein structure. *Proc. natn. Acad. Sci. U.S.A.* **80**, 7395.

De Kretser, T. A., Crumpton, M. J., Bodmer, J. G. & Bodmer, W. F. (1982) Two-dimensional gel analysis of the polypeptides precipitated by a polymorphic HLA-DR1, 2, w6 monoclonal antibody: evidence for a third locus. *Eur. J. Immunol.* **12**, 600.

De Mars, R., Chang, C. C., Marrari, M., Duquesnoy, R. J., Noreen, H., Segall, M. & Bach, F. H. (1983) Dissociation in expression of MB1/MT1 and DR1 alloantigens in mutants of a lymphoblastoid cell-line. *J. Immunol.* **131(3)**, 1318.

Hedrick, S. M., Nielsen, E. A., Kavaler, J., Cohen, I. E. & Davis, M. M. (1984) Sequence relationships between putative T-cell receptor polypeptides and immunoglobulins. *Nature (Lond.)*, **308**, 153.

Jones, P. P., Murphy, D. B. & McDevitt, H. O. (1978) Two-gene control of the expression of a murine Ia antigen. *J. exp. Med.* **148**, 925.

Kissmeyer-Nielsen, F., ed. (1975) *Histocompatibility Testing 1975. Report of the Sixth International Histocompatibility Workshop and Conference.* Munksgaard, Copenhagen.

W. Bodmer et al.

Larhammar, D., Schenning, L., Gustafsson, K., Wiman, K., Claesson, L., Rask, L. & Peterson, P. A. (1982) Complete amino acid sequence of an HLA-DR antigen-like β chain as predicted from the nucleotide sequence: similarities with immunoglobulins and HLA-A, -B, and -C antigens. *Proc. natn. Acad. Sci. U.S.A.* **79**, 3687.

Larhammar, D., Hyldig-Nielsen, J. J., Servenius, B., Andersson, G., Rask, L. & Peterson, P. A. (1983) Exon–intron organisation and complete nucleotide sequence of a human major histocompatibility antigen DCβ gene. *Proc. natn. Acad. Sci. U.S.A.* **80**, 7313.

Lee, J. S., Trowsdale, J. & Bodmer, W. F. (1982a) cDNA clones coding for the heavy chain of human HLA-DR antigen. *Proc. natn. Acad. Sci. U.S.A.* **79**, 545.

Lee, J. S., Trowsdale, J., Travers, P. J., Carey, J., Grosveld, F., Jenkins, J. & Bodmer, W. F. (1982b) Sequence of an HLA-DR α-chain cDNA clone and intron–exon organisation of the corresponding gene. *Nature (Lond.)*, **229**, 750.

Lee, J. A., Trowsdale, J., Travers, P. & Bodmer, W. F. (1983) Molecular analysis of the HLA-D region genes. *Human Immunol.* **8**, 105.

Long, E. L., Wake, C. T., Gorski, J. & Mach, B. (1983) Complete sequence of an HLA-DR β-chain deduced from a cDNA clone and identification of multiple non-allelic DR β-chain genes. *EMBO J.* **2**(3), 389.

Mostov, K. E., Friedlander, M. & Blobel, G. (1984) The receptor for transepithelial transport of IgA and IgM contains multiple immunoglobulin-like domains. *Nature (Lond.)*, **308**, 37.

Owen, M. J., Kissonerghis, A. M., Lodish, H. F. & Crumpton, M. J. (1981) Biosynthesis and maturation of HLA-DR antigens *in vivo*. *J. biol. Chem.* **256**, 8987.

Rudd, C. E., Bodmer, J. G., Bodmer, W. F. & Crumpton, M. J. (1984) HLA-D Region antigen associated invariant polypeptides as revealed by 2-D gel analysis: glycosylation and structural inter-relationships. *J. biol. Chem.* (in press).

Shackelford, D. A., Kaufman, J. F., Korman, A. J. & Strominger, J. L. (1982) HLA-DR antigens–structure, separation of sub-populations gene cloning and function. *Immunol. Rev.* **66**, 133.

Shaw, S., Kavathas, P., Pollack, M. A., Charmot, D. & Mawas, C. (1981) Family studies define a new histocompatibility locus, SB, between HLA-DR and GLO. *Nature (Lond.)*, **293**, 745.

Spielman, R. S., Lee, J., Bodmer, W. F., Bodmer, J. G. & Trowsdale, J. (1984) Six HLA-D α chain genes on human chromosome 6: polymorphisms and associations of DCα-related sequences with DR types. *Proc. natn. Acad. Sci. U.S.A.* **81**, 3461.

Steinmetz, M. & Hood, L. (1983) Genes of the major histocompatibility complex in mouse and man. *Science*, **222**, 727.

Tosi, R., Tanigaki, N., Centis, D., Ferrara, G. B. & Pressman, D. (1978) Immunological dissection of human Ia molecules. *J. exp. Med.* **148**, 1592.

Travers, P., Blundell, T., Sternberg, M. J. E. & Bodmer, W. F. Structural and evolutionary analysis of HLA-D region products. *Nature (Lond.)*, **310**, 235.

Trowsdale, J., Kelly, A., Lee, J., Carson, S., Austin, P. & Travers, P. (1984b) A linkage map of two HLA-SBα and β genes: an intron in one of the SBβ genes contains a processed pseudogene. *Cell* (in press).

Trowsdale, J., Lee, J. & Bodmer, W. F. (1984a) Molecular genetics of the HLA region. In: *Genetical Analysis of the Cell Surface* (ed. P. Goodfellow), Vol. 16, 'Receptors and Recognition', p. 83. Chapman & Hall.

Trowsdale, J., Lee, J., Carey, J., Grosveld, F., Bodmer, J. & Bodmer, W. (1983) Sequences related to HLA-DRα chain on human chromosome 6: restriction enzyme polymorphism detected with DCα chain probes. *Proc. natn. Acad. Sci. U.S.A.* **80**, 1972.

Wake, C. T., Long, E. O. & Mach, B. (1982) Allelic polymorphism and complexity of the genes for HLA-DR β-chains—direct analysis by DNA-DNA hybridization. *Nature (Lond.)*, **300**, 372.

Williams, A. F. & Gagnon, J. (1982) Neuronal cell Thy-1 glycoprotein: homology with immunoglobulin. *Science*, **216**, 696.

Chapter 7
New perspectives in HLA and disease

J. Dausset & D. Cohen

Unité de Recherches sur les Maladies du Sang, INSERM U.93, Hôpital Saint Louis, 2 place du Dr Fournier, 75475 Paris cedex 10, France

Summary. Using HLA gene probes of class I, class II α and β DC [now renamed DQ], and various endonuclease restriction enzymes (Hind III, EcoRI, EcoRV, PvuII) on the DNA of 40 parents and their children, we found a high degree of polymorphism in class I and II β genes. In both, about half of the 15–20 bands are variable. Polymorphism is also present in the α gene, although apparently to a lesser extent. This polymorphism always segregates with HLA.

Phenotypic and genotypic studies were performed. In many instances, the variable fragment or allogenotope correlated strongly but not completely with alleles of the HLA-A, B or DR loci.

We can propose a model of the cluster of genes in the HLA-A region, based on the study of 80 haplotypes. The number of genes would be variable. Only one gene is predicted in the A9 haplotype; most of the others possess at least two genes, and in some rare haplotypes three genes have been detected.

For class II, the β DC probe seems to correlate with products from both the DR and the DC locus. Our results suggest that the DR7 determinant is encoded by a DC-like gene.

The practical implications of these data are two-fold.

1   HLA genotyping is possible, and useful in the case of non-HLA expression on the cell surface, such as in the bare lymphocytic syndrome (two such cases are reported), and for the prenatal diagnosis of HLA-linked diseases such as the 21-OH deficiency.

2   HLA and disease associations will greatly benefit from these new techniques. New polymorphic markers will be found, closer to the susceptibility and resistance genes, and new diseases will be associated with these new polymorphisms.

In juvenile insulin-dependent diabetes, it was observed that the rare DR2 patients do not possess a β DC EcoRI 2·2 kb fragment which is almost always present in normal DR2 controls ($P = 10^{-5}$). This fragment is also present in Wolfram syndrome and multiple sclerosis patients. Another allogenotope, β DC PvuII, 4·0 kb, was also significantly less frequent in DR3 patients than in controls ($P = 2.10^{-2}$).

A β DC BamHI 12 kb fragment was found more frequently in multiple sclerosis patients than in controls (four times versus eight times in controls: not significant).

The future of this new technology in preventive medicine is discussed.

Introduction

The discovery of the H-2 antigens by Peter Gorer has opened up a new field of research and knowledge which has not stopped expanding over the years and which has revealed an extraordinary wealth of information. The description of the major histocompatibility complex (MHC) first in the mouse, then in man, immediately provided significant new applications in the field of public health. Organ and bone marrow transplantations were the first to be explored. Thousands of patients have already benefited from this breakthrough in knowledge and many others will in the future. The numerous diseases associated or linked to HLA have important implications in preventive medicine, and in the future these implications will be considerably greater thanks to modern methods of investigation, particularly molecular biology with which we are now able to reach the gene level where the actual cause of susceptibility or resistance to disease lies.

In view of the DNA polymorphism detected by endonuclease restriction enzymes, it is now possible: (i) to find a polymorphic restriction site which is closer to the susceptibility or resistance gene than the classic markers known at present; (ii) to track down the gene(s) themselves; (iii) to track down the *non*-HLA genes present in the HLA complex which could be responsible for diseases associated with or linked to HLA.

We used the Southern blotting technique in which the various fragments of DNA, obtained after dissection by several restriction enzymes at specific DNA sequences, are distributed in order of their size by electrophoresis. A radioactive HLA probe will hybridize only the HLA genes, all of which have a great nucleotide homology. The hybridization is revealed by autoradiography.

The first finding is that a large number of fragments hybridize with the class I probe (provided by Sood, Pereira & Weissman, 1981). Fifteen to 20 bands are visible per individual (Fig. 7.1), but it should not be forgotten that all human individuals are heterozygous and that the degree of stringency exercised in the conditions of hybridization influences the

J. Dausset & D. Cohen

Class I pB7 EcoR Ⅴ

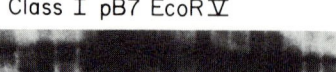

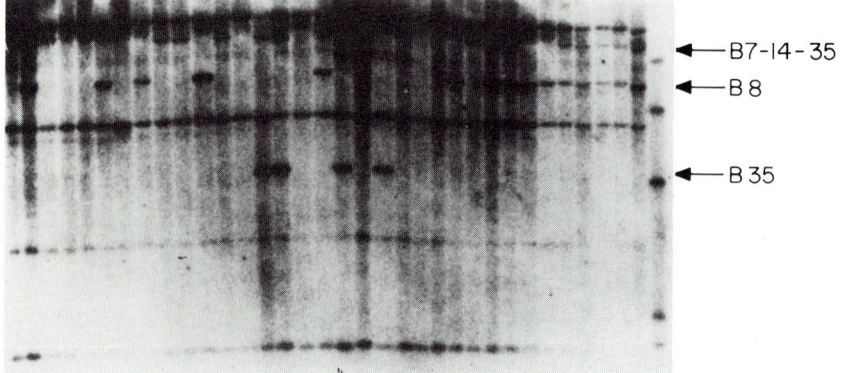

◄── B7-14-35
◄── B8

◄── B 35

Fig. 7.1. Southern blotting of DNA of 35 unrelated individuals digested with EcoR V and probed with class I cDNA. The polymorphism corresponding to B7, B8 and Bw35 are marked with *arrows*.

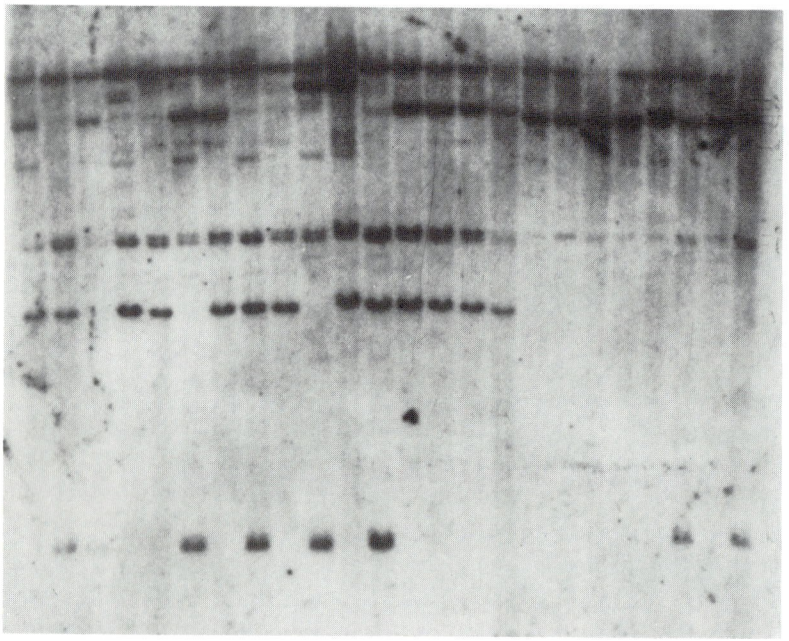

Fig. 7.2. Southern blotting of DNA of 24 unrelated individuals digested with EcoR V and probed with class II β DC cDNA.

number of bands. Moreover, a gene can be represented by two bands if the cutting is intragenic.

The second important observation is the frequent polymorphism of these fragments. We shall call them 'allogenotopes' instead of 'polymorphic fragments' which is meaningless.

With a β DC probe (provided by Larhammar *et al.*, 1982), we usually find 10–20 bands which also exhibit a distinct polymorphism (Fig. 7.2). With the α DC probe (provided by Auffray *et al.*, 1983), the number of bands is obviously less (three or four) but the polymorphism is nevertheless present (Fig. 7.3).

Class II α HIND III

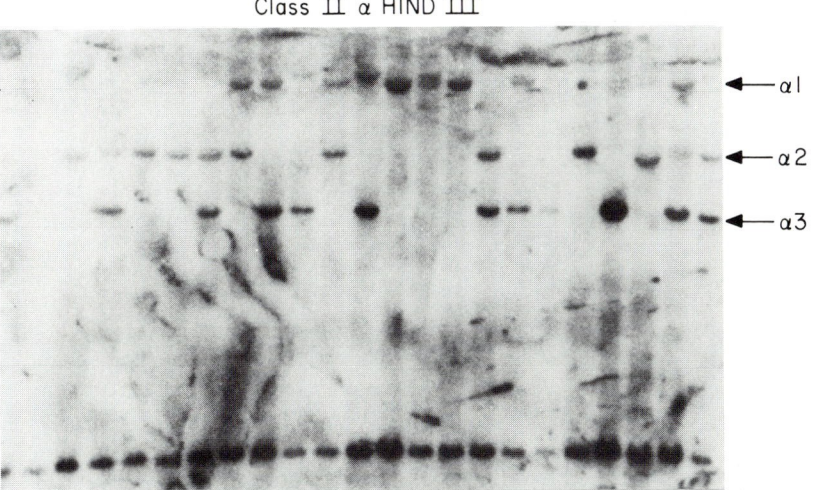

Fig. 7.3. Southern blotting of DNA of 24 unrelated individuals digested with Hind III and probed with class II β DC cDNA. The polymorphic fragments are marked with *arrows*.

These observations confirm and extend the polymorphisms reported by Ascanio *et al.* (1982) and Auffray *et al.* (1983) for class I, Trowsdale *et al.* (1983) for class II α DR, Wake, Long & Mach (1982) for class II β DR, Owerbach *et al.* (1983b) for β DC, and by one of the present authors (D.C.) in Roux-Dosseto *et al.* (1983) for β SB [now renamed DP].

The third interesting finding was that the DNA polymorphism always segregated with HLA (Fig. 7.4). Up till now, any HLA fragment of either class I or II has segregated with HLA, indicating that there is probably no polymorphic gene of the same structure outside the HLA complex.

Segregation of BglI class I α allogenotopes

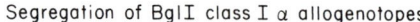
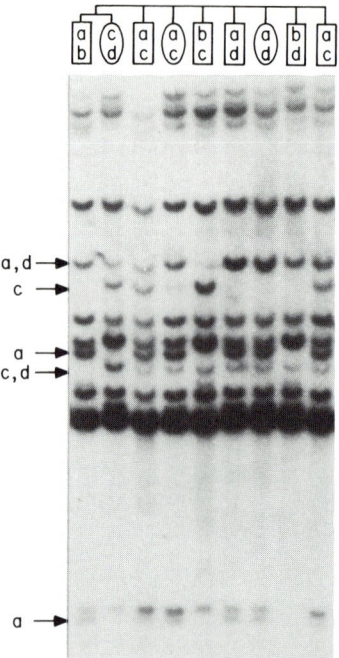

Fig. 7.4. Southern blotting of DNA of a family with Bgl I and probed with class I cDNA. The fragments marked by arrows segregate with the HLA haplotypes of the parents (a, b, c, d).

With this new tool it is possible, with only one enzyme or with several, to construct new allelic series, associated or not associated with the HLA series already known, thus providing new markers of the HLA complex. Such new allelic series are now emerging. But we wish to point out here the numerous and sometimes very strong correlations which exist between some of these fragments and the known HLA alleles. There are three possibilities in this respect: (i) that the HLA gene is completely included in the fragment; (ii) only part of the gene is included in the fragment; (iii) the fragment contains a gene, or part of a gene, in linkage disequilibrium with the expressed gene.

Genetic analysis of normal individuals

A systematic study based on these hypotheses was carried out on a panel of 40 normal, non-related parents and their children.

Phenotypic study with a class I probe and Hind III

We observed three allogenotypes (Fig. 7.5). The first one, of 4·8 kb, correlated with A1 plus A11, and the second, of 5·0 kb, correlated with A9 (Aw24 and Aw23), as shown in a more extensive study (in preparation) with two well-known cross-reactions. This fact should have some

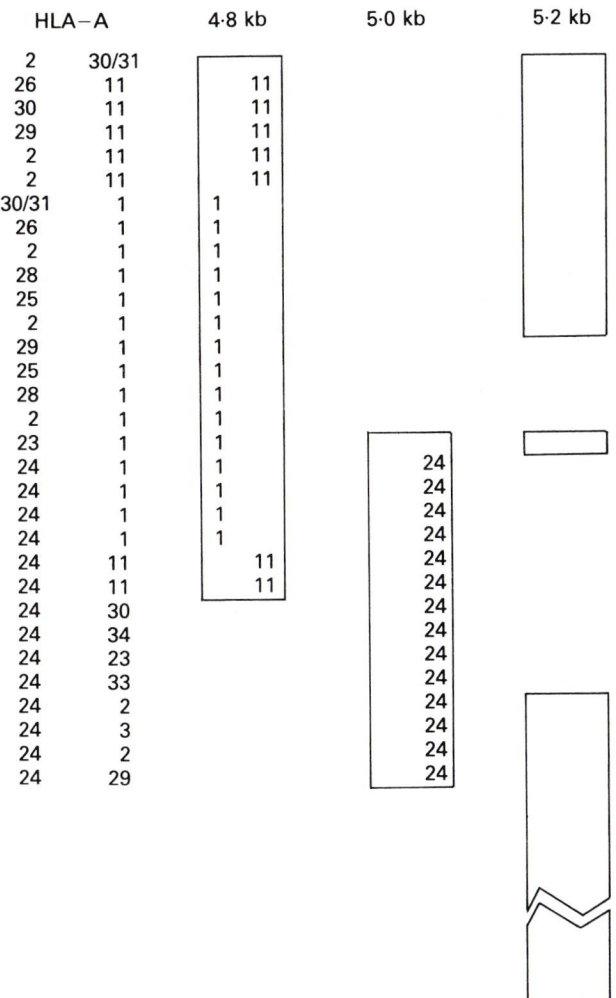

Fig. 7.5. Phenotypic distribution of three polymorphic class I restriction fragments in 68 normal unrelated Caucasians, showing correlations with HLA alleles.

biological or evolutionary significance. It could be explained if either the same polymorphic site were intragenic in the two genes, or if this polymorphic site were situated on a gene in close linkage with the two genes encoding the cross-reacting products. A third allogenotope of 5·2 kb was found in most of the individuals tested, presenting a contrasting distribution with the first two allogenotopes.

Genotypic study with a class I probe and Hind III

Next we tested the children of these 40 parents, and deduced 80 haplotypes. The clearest analysis of the correlations was found with the HLA-A alleles. In Fig. 7.6, the HLA antigens are listed vertically with an equal length for each (their respective percentages are given in the left-hand column). Here again, the previous three allogenotopes (4·8, 5·0 and 5·2 kb) have the same correlations. Three other allogenotopes were found: a 7·0 kb fragment present in all A1, A11, A3, A10, A28, A2 individuals and in some Aw19 individuals. The other Aw19 individuals possessed a 7·4 kb fragment and a 4·9 kb fragment. It is evident (i) that fragments 5·0, 4·8, 5·2 and 7·4 behave as an allelic series; (ii) that the 4·9 fragment does not fit into this allelic series; (iii) that the 7·0 fragment 'includes' completely both the 4·8 and 5·2 fragments.

From a restriction map of the HLA-A clones published by Lemonnier *et al.* (1983) (clones from an A3, A9 individual), it is clear that the 5·0 kb, 5·2 kb and 7·0 kb fragments include a complete gene. The 4·8 kb fragment hybridized with 5′ and 3′ class I probes containing sequences of both ends of an HLA gene. Thus, this fragment probably also contains a complete gene.

With this information in mind, we constructed a model of the HLA-A gene cluster (Fig. 7.7). In the haplotype bearing A9, Jordan *et al.* (1983) found only one gene. Our results with Hind III and also EcoRV (data not shown) suggest the same interpretations. The other haplotypes carry at least two genes detected by the 4·8 and 7·0 kb fragments for A1 and A11 haplotypes, or detected by the 5·2 and 7·0 kb fragments for the A2, A3, A10, A28 haplotypes and part of Aw19. It is important to note that the 5·0 kb fragment expressed A9 (Lemonnier *et al.*, 1983) and that the 4·8 kb fragment expressed A11 (data not shown).

Another two genes (4·9 kb and 7·4 kb), for which we do not know the allelic correspondence with the two previous loci, are found in some other Aw19 haplotypes. Finally, only three of the 80 haplotypes contain three genes detected by the 5·2, 7·0 and 4·9 kb fragments. The 4·9 kb fragments

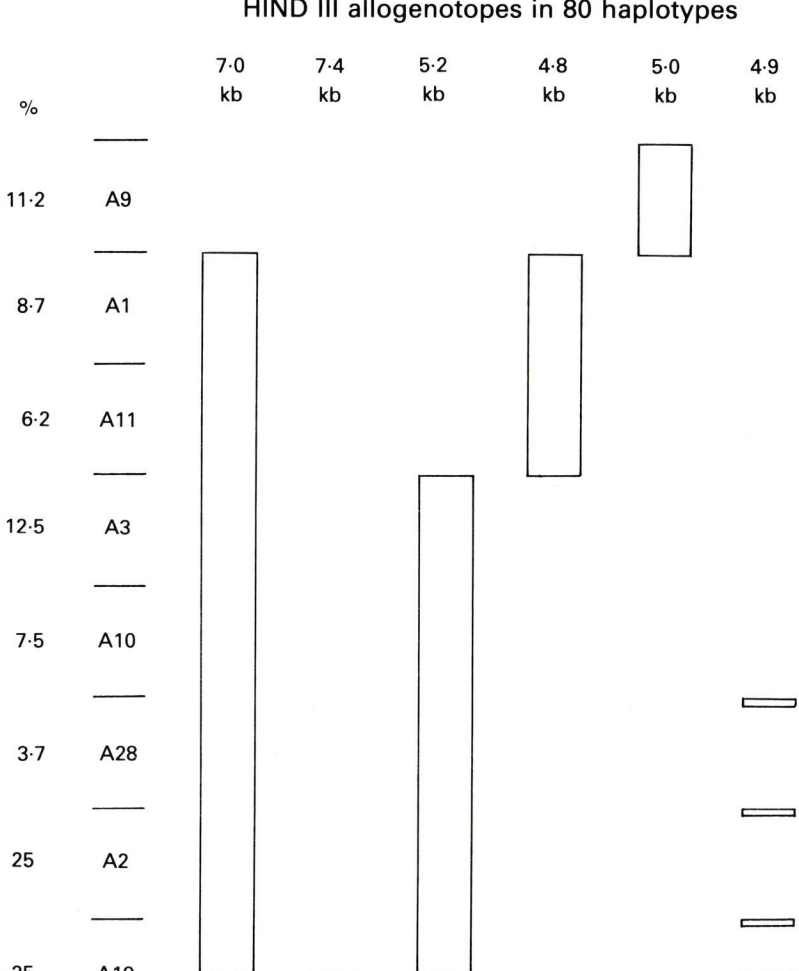

Fig. 7.6. Genotypic distribution of six polymorphic class I restriction fragments in 80 haplotypes deduced from normal unrelated Caucasians, showing correlations with HLA-A alleles. For clarity, each allele is represented by the same length, but their respective percentages are given on the left.

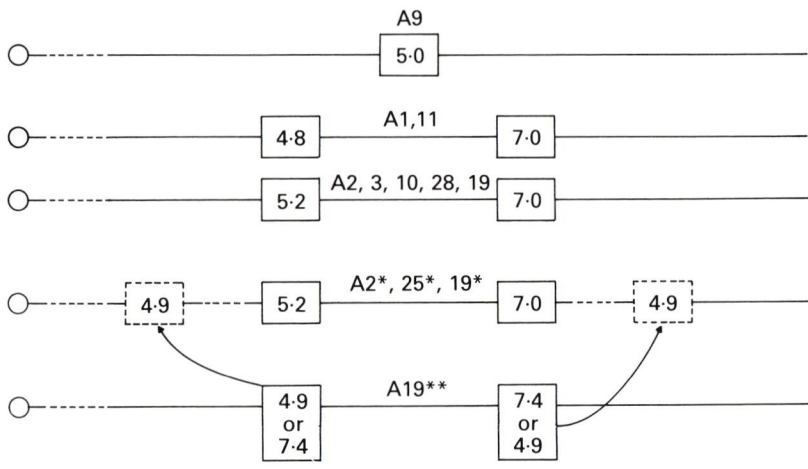

Fig. 7.7. An evolutionary model for the HLA-A region, based on 80 haplotypes. Each line represents the small arm of the sixth chromosome, with the centromere (0) on the left. The position of the 4·8, 5·2 and 7·0 kb fragments is determined, while that of the 4·9 and 7·4 kb is not. * One haplotype each. ** Three haplotypes.

could have been introduced in these rare haplotypes by unequal crossing-over.

We suggest that the HLA-A gene cluster may contain a variable number of loci, perhaps only one for the A9 haplotype, but often at least two and occasionally three. This may possibly reflect the expansion–contraction phenomenon of the genome. This is of course only a model, which will have to be confirmed by a restriction map of these clusters.

Phenotypic study with a class I probe and the enzymes Hind III and EcoRV

The same approach was taken with the HLA-B locus. Without going into detail about the correlation shown in Fig. 7.8, it is obvious that strong correlations exist between Bw35 and the EcoRV 4·6 kb fragment, between B15 and the Hind III 2·3 kb fragment, between B8 and the EcoRV 8·6 kb fragment (Cann *et al.*, 1983), and between B40 and the Hind III 10·0 kb fragment (Cohen & Dausset, 1983; Cohen *et al.*, 1983). It is evident (i) that there are some exceptions but these always follow the same direction, that is to say, all individuals carrying serologically detected antigens always possess the fragment, but the reverse does not apply; (ii) that the fragment correlating with Bw35 is completely 'included' in the larger EcoRV 13·4 fragment.

HLA−B allogenotopes in controls

HLA−B		EcoRV 13·4 kb	4·6 kb	HIND III 2·3 kb	EcoRV 8·6 kb	HIND III 10·0 kb
7	35	7 35	35			
12	35	35	35			
39	35	35	35			
35	35	35 35	35 35			
27	35	35	35			
38	35	5 35	35			
22	35	35	35			
5	35	5 35	35			
27	35	35	35	•		•
39	55					
44	38					
18	40					40
7	60	7				60
7	38	7				
7	39	7				
7	12	7				
7	51	7 5				
7	15	7		•		•
7	49	7				
7	14	7 14				
18	14	14				
12	14	14				
18	14	14				
27	14	14		•		•
51	18	5				
5	17	5				
51	8	5			8	
5	8	5			8	
14	8	14			8	
7	8	7			8	
7	18	7				
52	60					
18	44					
18	60					60
13	13					
15	13			15		
62	13			15		
15	61			15		
15	15			15 15		
15	12			15		
63	44			15		
15	27			15		
15	12			15		
15	8			15	8	
51	8				8	
39	8				8	
18	8				8	
12	8				8	
44	8				8	
18	8				8	•
12	8			•	8	•
22	8			•	8	•
12	60					60
22	60					60

12 others without B5, 7, 8, 14, 15, 60

Fig. 7.8. Phenotypic distribution of five polymorphic class I restriction fragments in 66 normal unrelated Caucasians, showing correlations with HLA-B alleles. (•), Not done.

Phenotypic study with class II α DC probe and Hind III

A good correlation was observed with the known DR alleles: (i) fragment 'a' (5·5 kb) is present in all DR4 and DR7 (i.e. MT3) individuals; (ii) fragment 'b' (7·0 kb) is present in all DR3 and DR5 (i.e. MT2) individuals; (iii) fragment 'c' (9.5 kb) is present in all DR1 and DR2 (i.e. MT1) individuals (Fig. 7.9). Is the serologically defined MT series therefore the reflection of α chain polymorphism (Fig. 7.10)?

HIND III DCα allogenotopes in

		Controls				IDD			
SB	DR	a	b	c	other DR	a	b	c	other DR
						4	+		1
						4			−
	4 3	4			3	4	3		
4 *	4 −	4			−	4	3		
2 3	4 −	4			−	4	3		
	4 7	4/7				4	3		
	− 7	7	+		−	4	3		
	3 7	7	?		3?	4	3		
	3 7	7	3			4	3		
	4 4	4/4	+			4	3		
4 *	4 5	4	5			+	3/5		
	4 5	4	5			+	3/5		
	4 1	4	?			4			
4 5	3 1	+		1	3	4		+	
	5 1		5	1				2	
3 4	5 1		5	1			?	+	4/−
	5 3		5/3				+	2	−
3 4	5 *		5*				3	1	−
4 *	5 *		5*				3	+	
4 *	3 −		3		−		3	1	
	3 *		3*					2/1	
	2 2			2/2					
4 *	2 6			2	6				
5 *	2 *			2*					
Interpretation : MT		3	2	1		MT 3	2	1	
DR		4,7	3,5	1,2		4	3,5	1,2	

Fig. 7.9. Phenotypic distribution of three polymorphic class II α DC Hind III restriction fragments in 22 normal unrelated Caucasians and 20 IDD patients, showing correlations with HLA-DR and MT specificities. * Possibly homozygote. (−), Blank.

Phenotypic study with class II β DC probe and BgII

Fragment 'a' correlates strongly with DR1; fragment 'e' correlates with DR4 and DR5, i.e. MB3; fragments 'f' and 'h' correlate with DR3 and DR7, i.e. MB2. Two other fragments, 'b' and 'g' do not correlate with any known alleles (Fig. 7.11).

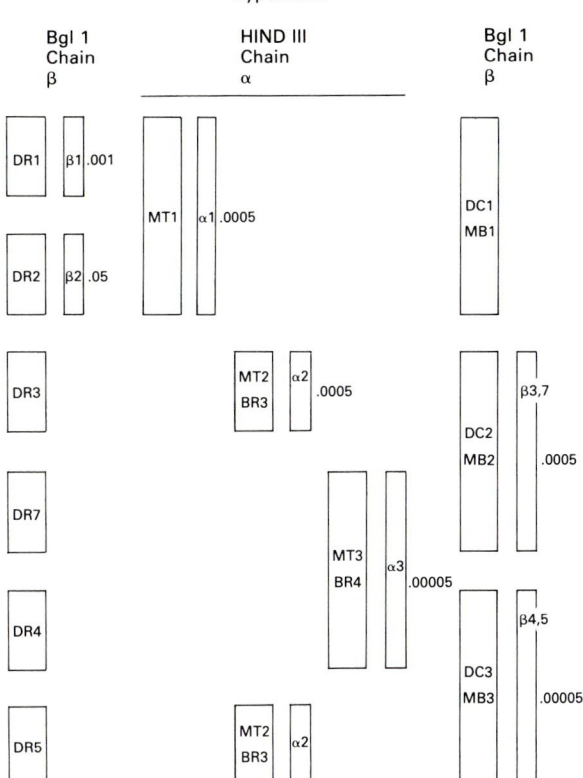

Fig. 7.10. Correlations obtained with polymorphic class II α and β fragments and DR and MT specificities. A striking correlation was obtained between three α DC fragments and MT1, MT2 and MT3, and between two β DC fragments and MB2 and MB3.

Genotypic studies with class II β DC probe and two enzymes (Hind III and EcoRV)

Seventy haplotypes were deduced from family studies. With Hind III, four allogenotopes present a strong correlation with DR alleles. The 12·6 kb fragment correlates with DR3, with one exception. The 13·8 kb fragment correlates with DR7, with one exception (DR3). The 3·6 kb fragment correlates with DR5, but with two exceptions (DR4 and DR−). These three fragments show allelic behaviour. On the other hand, the 6·9 kg fragment correlates with DC1 alleles, comprising DR1, DR2, DRw6 and DR− (Fig. 7.12).

J. Dausset & D. Cohen

Bgl DC β Allogenotopes in controls

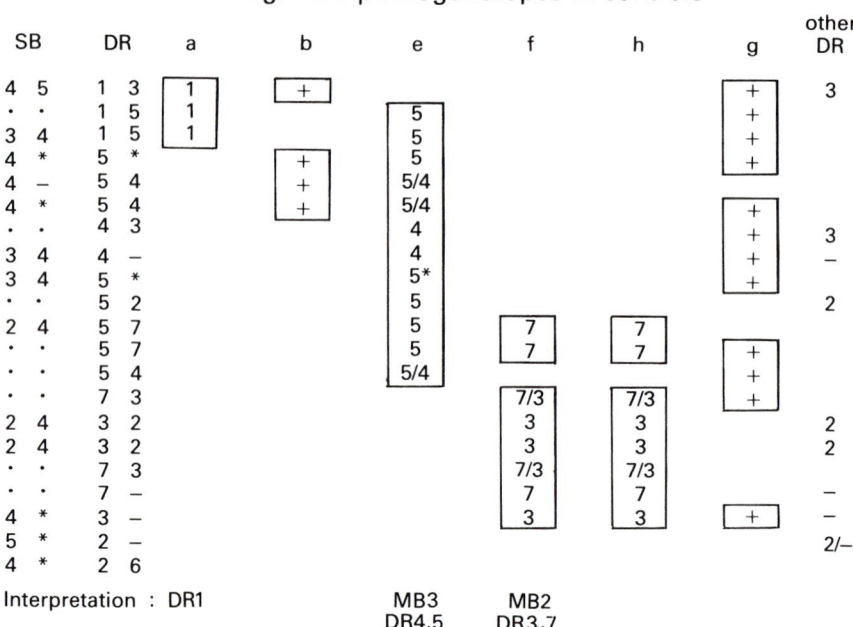

Fig. 7.11. Phenotypic distribution of six polymorphic class II β DC Bgl I restriction fragments in 21 normal unrelated caucasoid individuals showing correlation with HLA-DR and MB specificities. * Possibly homozygote. (•), Not done. (–), Blank.

An analogous picture was obtained when the same haplotype study was done with EcoRV. Here also, two fragments correlate with the DR alleles: DR7 for fragment 'b' (2·5 kb); DR5, DRw8, DRw9 and five other non-DR5, w8 or w9 alleles for fragment 'e' (18 kb). Three other fragments, 'h' (6·8 kb), 'i' (5·2 kb) and 'j' (2·6 kb) detect various portions of DC1 (Fig. 7.13).

It is remarkable that all these fragments are detected by a DC probe under non-stringent conditions of washing. However the bands corresponding to DC1 remain under stringent conditions of hybridization, as does the band correlating with DR7 when using both enzymes. This suggests that DR7 might be encoded by a DC-like allele which could map either at the DC or DR locus. This last observation could correspond to the absence of reactivity of DR7 products with many monomorphic monoclonal anti-DR antibodies (P. Ivanyi, personal communication).

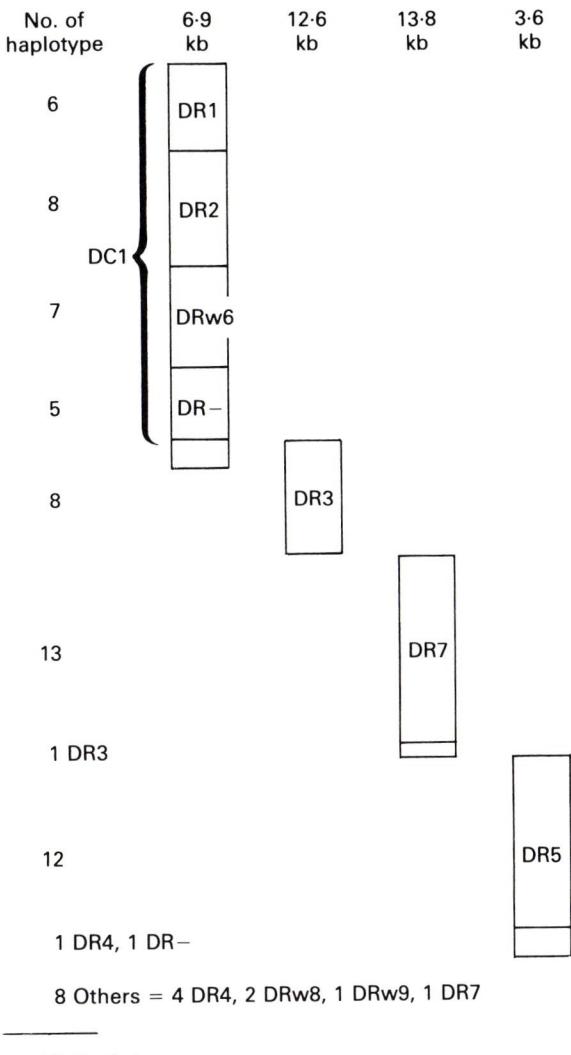

HIND III β DC allogenotopes correlate with DC and DR in 70 haplotypes

70 Haplotypes

Fig. 7.12. Genotypic distribution of four polymorphic class II β DC Hind III restriction fragments in 70 haplotypes deduced from normal caucasoid families showing correlation with HLA-DR and DC specificities.

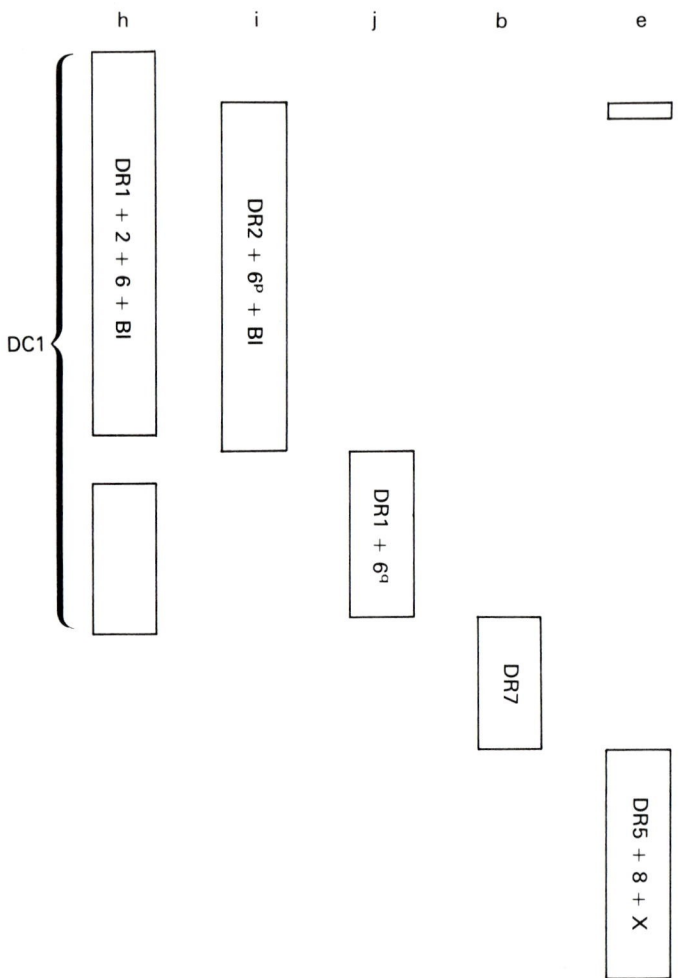

Fig. 7.13. Genotypic distribution of five polymorphic class II β DC EcoR V restriction fragments in 70 haplotypes deduced from normal caucasoid families showing correlation with HLA-DR and DC specificities (h = 6·8 kb, i = 5·2 kb, j = 2·6 kb, b = 25 kb, e = 18 kb).

Practical implications

HLA genotyping with DNA fragments in the case of non-expressed HLA products

It is now possible, without having any knowledge of the products, to genotype an individual with the exclusive use of DNA allogenotypes (Marcadet *et al.*, in preparation). This is particularly useful when the molecules are not expressed on the cell surface, such as in the bare lymphocytic syndrome and in some severe immunodeficiencies. In two such cases (kindly provided by Professor Griscelli), we were able to determine the HLA genotype of the patients, and in one case to designate the correct bone marrow donor.

In the first case (Fig. 7.14), the DNA haplotypes of both parents were deduced. The 'a' haplotype bears only one class I fragment (EcoRV, 13·4 kb), while the 'b' haplotype bears numerous fragments of both class I and II. The 'a' and 'c' haplotypes are identical, which is not surprising since the parents are first cousins. The diseased child was found to be identical to the father, who was therefore chosen as the donor.

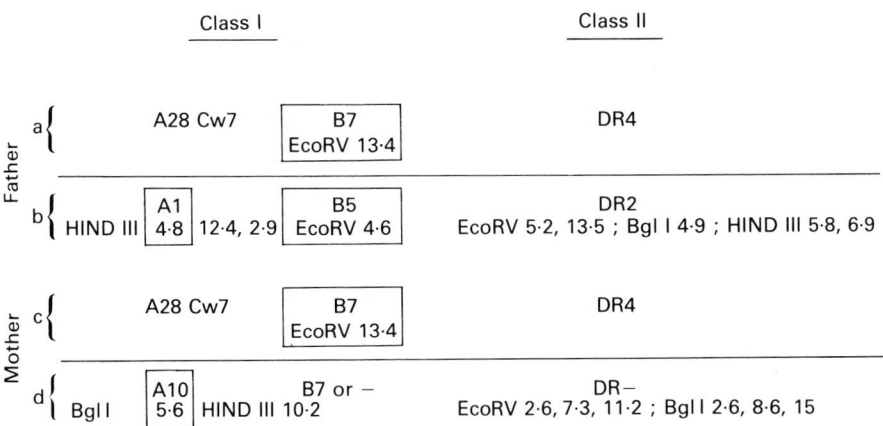

Fig. 7.14. In a first (LS) case with severe immunodeficiency, the four HLA haplotypes of the parents (a, b, c, d) were deduced from the DNA restriction fragments of the parents and a healthy child. For each haplotype are listed (*above*) the serologically defined antigens and (*below*) the DNA restriction fragments obtained with a class I probe (*left*) and class II β DC (*right*). The known correlation between serologically defined antigen and a given restriction fragment are framed. Diseased child = bc (genetically identical to father). Healthy child = ac.

The second case (Fig. 7.15) is similar, but unfortunately the diseased child was found to be HLA-different from his siblings and bone marrow grafting was impossible. In both cases, the already known correlations with HLA alleles present in the parents' phenotypes were used to select the useful enzyme. Such correlations are of great help in interpreting the data.

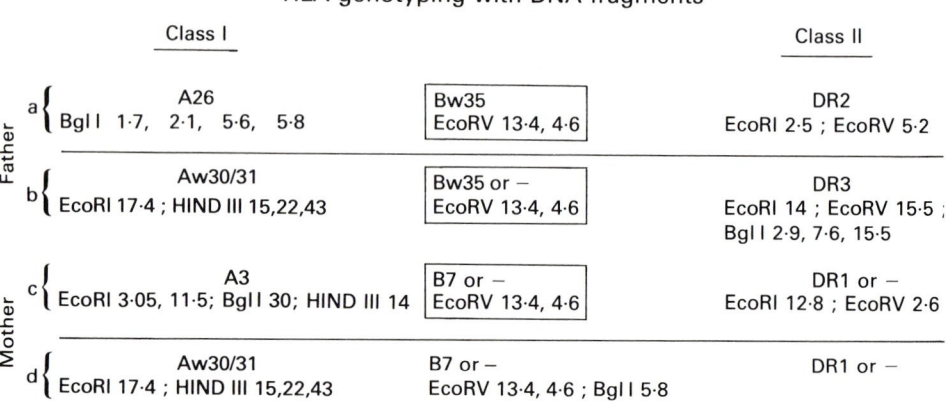

Fig. 7.15. Second case (RA) with severe immunodeficiency (same legend as Fig. 7.14). Diseased child = bc. Healthy child = ac.

HLA genotyping with DNA fragments for pre-natal diagnosis

At present, fibroblasts are taken by amniocentesis at the 20th week of pregnancy, but not without some degree of risk to the foetus and, in the case of abortion, with severe psychological consequences for the mother. For DNA genotyping, biopsy of chorionic villi can be performed as early as the 6th–8th week, with a much lower risk for both the mother and the foetus.

HLA and disease associations

Juvenile insulin-dependent diabetes (IDD)

(i) Immunogenetically, IDD is characterized by a much stronger association of heterozygous DR3/DR4 than of DR3 or DR4 alone, suggesting that both haplotypes contribute to the susceptibility; (ii) resistance is associated with DR2; (iii) the excess of affected HLA-identical siblings (59% instead of the expected 25%) is another indication that both are important; (iv) in Caucasians, three haplotypes in strong linkage disequilibrium are frequently implicated and, remarkably, all of them carry a deficient C4 allele, either at the C4A or the C4B locus.

We studied 24 diabetic patients and the same number of normal individuals: (i) with an α DC probe and Hind III enzyme, it was clear (Fig. 7.9) that approximately the same correlation pattern was observed in both groups; (ii) when using a β DC probe and EcoRI, we observed that a 2·2 kb fragment gave a peculiar distribution. It was equally rare in non-DR2 controls and patients (Fig. 7.16). However, this 2·2 kb fragment was present in all but one of the DR2 controls and absent in each of the seven rare DR2 patients tested ($P = 5 \times 10^{-5}$). It was later found in one non-DR2 patient, indicating that this polymorphic site (or sites) is not responsible for protection. This band remains under stringent conditions of washing, suggesting that it might correspond to a DC gene (Cohen *et al.*, 1984). The lack of this 2·2 kb fragment in DR2 IDD patients should be compared to that in the study of Bach *et al.* (1982), who stated that none of the five Caucasian DR2 patients they tested possessed the Dw2 or Dw12 specificity (out of 63 controls, 56 are Dw2 or Dw12). However, one black DR2 patient was Dw2. Work is in progress to establish whether or not Bach's observation and our own have the same genetic background. It will also have to be established whether DR2 patients belong in particular to one or other of the new serological splits of DR2.

In 18 matched DR3 patients, a β DC PvuII fragment was found only once, compared with seven times in controls ($P = 2.10^{-2}$) (Fig. 7.17). Our results are in agreement with those of Owerbach *et al.* (1983a) who found that in DR4 patients, there was a decrease of the BamHI 2·7 kb fragment ($P = 3.10^{-3}$) and an increase of the Pst 18 kb fragment ($P = 1.10^{-3}$). With the exception of the last fragment, all the others present a decreased frequency. This might suggest the lack of a gene, or genes, which could be involved in the resistance to diabetes.

Is the same susceptibility or resistance gene carried by the DR3 and DR4 haplotypes, or are there two different genes in the two haplotypes? Molecular biology will be of great help in solving this important problem, and in understanding the physio-pathology of the disease.

Random controls		Matched controls		IDD		Wolfram	
DR	RI 2·2 kb	DR	RI 2·2 kb	DR	RI 2·2 kb	DR	RI 2·2 kb
1,4	−	2,1	+	2,1	−	F 2,4	+
2,5	+	2,1	−	2,1	−	M 1,5	−
2,5	+	2,3	+	2,3	−	C1 1,4	−
2,4	+	2,3	+	2,3	−	C2 2,5	+
2,3	+	2,3	+	2,3	−	C3 2,5	+
3,7	−	2,4	+	2,4	−		
3,7	−	2,7	+	2,7	−		
3,7	−						
3,3	−						
3,5	−			4,7	−		
3*	−			4,3	−		
3,−	+			4,3	−		
7,7	−			4,3	−		
5,7	−			4,3	−		
7,−	−			4,3	−		
4,4	−			4,3	−		
4,−	+			4,3	−		
4,−	−			4,3	−		
4*	−			4,3	−		
4,5	−			4,3	−		
5,−	−			4,3	−		
5*	−			4,1	−		
				5,3	−		
Selected DR2 homozygous				4,−	+		
				1,3	−		
2,2	+			3,5	−		
2,2	+			4,3	−		
2,2	+			3,6	−		
2,2	+			7,6	−		
2,2	+						

Fig. 7.16. Distribution of EcoRI 2·2 kb β DC fragment in insulin-dependent diabetes (IDD) and in one family of Wolfram Syndrome. Note that this allogenotope is rare in non-DR2 controls, present in all but one DR2 control, absent in the seven IDD patients, while it was found in all but one of the 15 MS DR2 patients tested (not shown in this table). * Possibly homozygous. F = father; M = mother; C1, C2, C3 = affected siblings. RI = EcoRI.

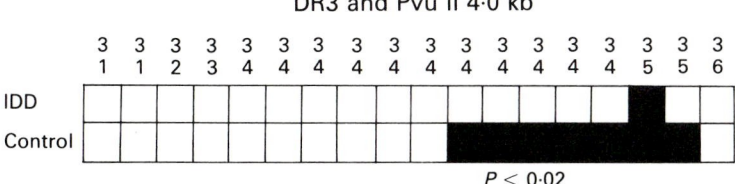

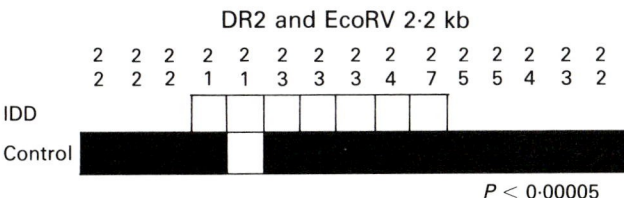

Fig. 7.17. β DC DNA restriction fragments differentiate between HLA-DR3 and DR2 individuals in insulin-dependent diabetes (IDD). DR3 and DR2 IDD patients were DR-matched with normal controls and the β DC restriction fragments were compared.

Wolfram syndrome

Before leaving the subject of diabetes, it must be noted that in one family of Wolfram syndrome, which is a particular form of familial diabetes, possibly associated with DR2 (Deschamps *et al.*, 1983; Monson & Boucher, 1983), the EcoRI β DC 2·2 kb fragment was present, thus emphasizing (if necessary) the heterogeneity of the disease.

Multiple sclerosis (MS)

Twenty-four MS patients and the same number of DR-matched controls, as well as 45 random controls (Fig. 7.18) were studied. A BamHI β DC fragment was found 11 times in the random controls (mostly associated with DR4) and four times in the matched controls, as compared with eight times in the MS patients. Of these eight patients, four were DR2. However, this difference is not significant. The relevant risk for DR2 individuals is 4·0 in the general population, rising to 8·8 for those who are both DR2- and band 12 kb-positive, and 7·2 for those who are both DC1- and band 12 kb-positive.

The MS patients were also tested with EcoRI and β DC probes. All

Random controls				Matched controls		MS	
DR	BHI 12 kb	DR	BHI 12 kb	DR	BHI 12 kb	DR	BHI 12 kb
1,–	–	4,–	[+]	1,2	–	1,2	–
1,2	–	4,2	+	1,2	–	1,2	–
1,2	–	4,5	+	1,2	–	1,2	–
1,5	–	4,5	+	1,3	–	1,3	[+]
1,6	–	4,7	+	2,3	–	2,3	–
1,6	[+]	4,7	[+]	2,3	–	2,3	–
1,7	–	4,6	–	2,4	–	2,4	[+]
2,–	–	5,–	[+]	2,5	–	2,5	–
2,3	–	5,–	[+]	2,5	–	2,5	[+]
2,3	–	5,–	–	2,5	–	2,5	–
2,3	–	5,–	–	2,6	–	2,6	[+]
2,3	–	5,–	–	2,6	–	2,6	[+]
2,5	–	5,1	–	2,7	–	2,7	–
2,6	–	5,7	–	2,7	–	2,7	–
2,7	–	5,8	–	2,–	[+]	2,*	–
2,7	–	6,6	–	2,–	[+]	2,–	–
3,5	–	7,–	–	3,5	[+]	3,5	–
3,5	–	7,–	–	3,7	–	3,7	[+]
3,6	–	7,*	–	3,–	–	3,*	–
3,7	[+]	7,6	–	4,7	[+]	4,7	[+]
3,–	[+]	7,7	–	4,7	–	4,7	–
4.–	–	8,–	–	5,–	–	5,*	–
		9,–	–	6,–	–	6,*	[+]
				7,–	–	7,*	–

Fig. 7.18. Distribution of BamHI (BHI) 12 kb β DC in multiple sclerosis (MS) patients. * Possibly heterozygous.

but one of 15 DR2 patients possess the 2·2 kb fragment. It can be said, regarding the presence or absence of this band, that susceptibility to MS is found in both categories of DR2 (since the proportion of DR2-positive and -negative bands is the same as in the controls), while resistance to diabetes seems to be specific only to those who carry this fragment.

Conclusion

Human genetics is entering a new era of its history, thanks to molecular biology which enables us to work at the gene level. At present more than 50 human diseases, most of them of unknown aetiology, are either associated with or linked to HLA. The biochemical basis of these correlations can now be elucidated, thanks to the extraordinary polymorphism of the endonuclease restriction sites. It is amazing that with only a few enzymes (three to five) and three HLA probes (class I, α II and β II), we have already been able to detect more than 100 polymorphic sites in the HLA complex. This reflects greater structural differences between alleles than was previously thought possible.

The first consequence of this polymorphism will probably be to refine the already known associations. More polymorphic markers, more closely associated with susceptibility or resistance, will be found and these will be a useful guide for clinicians. This will mark a new beginning for predictive, or even preventive medicine, in short for personalized medicine.

It is also probable that new diseases will be added to the list, particularly when these diseases are associated with a new DNA polymorphism which has *no* association with any of the classic HLA alleles.

Chromosome walking on the genome, from one overlapping fragment to another, will make it possible to explore the HLA complex section by section. At the beginning, the flanking regions of the HLA genes can be explored. This is how non-HLA were determined in the HLA-D region (Trowsdale *et al.*, personal communication). Subsequent exploration towards the centromere could have the ambitious aim of defining the human equivalent of the T system in the mouse, which may be responsible for spina bifida and associated disorders. However, the distance is probably too great. Exploration directed towards the telomere will be more realistic, since the human equivalent of the Qa-T1 region of the H-2 complex is close by and is still unexplored. This direction is interesting, because some weak associations are known between HLA-A alleles and malignant haemopoietic diseases (acute lymphocytic leukaemia with A2; Hodgkin's disease with A1).

Transfection will bring even more rewards. Gene cloning and its transfection enables us to study the biochemistry of the product, and hopefully, its function (either directly or indirectly), that is, after manipulation of the gene itself prior to transfection. The ultimate goal is to understand the physio-pathological mechanisms of these diseases and to identify accurately and characterize the gene or genes responsible for the diseases.

This will be a rather easy task in the monogenic diseases with full penetration, but most probably a difficult task in the polygenic diseases with weak penetration. Several different genes of the HLA complex could be involved either in a synergistic way (and the role played by class III genes, coding for defective complement factors, should not be underestimated), or in a complementary manner, possibly in transposition, which could be one explanation for the IDD situation.

Finally, following the recent discovery that HLA sequences are present in human T cell leukaemia virus (Clarke, Gelmann & Reitz, 1983), it seems an intriguing possibility to search in the patient's genome for insertions of some virus sequences close to the HLA genes.

With these new tools, the study of HLA and disease association will undoubtedly have important feedback in the understanding of normal processes, such as the normal immune response. However, prediction and understanding of the mechanisms is not enough. All this work should, and certainly will, lead to therapeutic advances, the most promising being the correction of metabolic disorders thanks to the transfer of cloned genes in somatic cells. HLA and other closely linked genes are good candidates. However, this new approach in modern medicine should be embarked upon with great care, bearing in mind the ethical considerations.

Acknowledgments

We would like to thank S. Weissman, C. Auffray, J. Strominger, D. Larhammar and P. Peterson for the generous gift of their probes; J. Hors, I. Deschamps (IDD patients), J. M. Degos, E. Schuller, A. Govaerts (MS patients) and C. Griscelli (bare lymphocyte syndrome) for their contributions to the study of diseases. We also express our gratitude to all the members of the team: O. Cohen, M. P. Font, I. Le Gall, A. Marcadet, C. Massart, M. Massé, E. Mornet, P. Paul and B. Sayagh, whose enthusiastic work made this presentation possible. We also thank E. May for editing and typing the manuscript.

References

Ascanio, L., Paul, P., Marcadet, A., Mahouy, G., Fradelizi, D., Cohen, D. & Dausset, J. (1982). Polymorphism des gènes HLA (I): mise en évidence d'une étroite corrélation entre des fragments d'ADN déterminés par l'enzyme de restriction BglI et des antigènes HLA de classe I. *C.R. Acad. Sci. (Paris)*, **295**, 433.

Auffray, C., Ben-nun, A., Roux-Dosseto, M., Germain, R. N., Seidman, J. G. & Strominger, J. L. (1983) Polymorphism and complexity of the human DC and murine Ia α chain genes. *EMBO J.* **2**, 121.

Bach, F. H., Segall, M., Rich, S. & Barbosa, S. (1982) HLA and susceptibility to type I diabetes. Hypothesis. *Tiss. Antigens*, **20**, 28.

Cann, H. M., Ascanio, L., Paul, P., Marcadet, A., Dausset, J. & Cohen, D. (1983) Polymorphic restriction endonuclease fragment segregates and correlates with the gene for HLA-B8. *Proc. natn. Acad. Sci. U.S.A.* **80**, 1665.

Clarke, M. F., Gelmann, E. P. & Reitz, M. S. (1983) Homology of Human T-cell leukaemia virus envelope gene with class I HLA gene. *Nature (Lond.)*, **305**, 60.

Cohen, D., Cohen, O., Massart, C., Lathrop, M., Descamps, I., Hors, J., Schuller, E. & Dausset, J. (1984) HLA class II β DC DNA restriction fragments differentiate among HLA-DR2 individuals in insulin-dependent diabetes and multiple sclerosis. *Proc. natn. Acad. Sci. U.S.A.* **81**, 1774.

Cohen, D. & Dausset, J. (1983) HLA genes polymorphism. In: *Progress in Immunology*, Vol. 5 (eds Y. Yamamura and T. Tada), p. 1. Academic Press.

Cohen, D., Paul, P., Font, M. P., Cohen, O., Sayagh, B., Marcadet, A., Busson, M., Mahouy, G., Cann, H. M. & Dausset, J. (1983) Analysis of HLA class I genes with restriction endonuclease fragments: implications for polymorphism of the human major histocompatibility complex. *Proc. natn. Acad. Sci. U.S.A.* **80**, 6289.

Deschamps, I., Lestradet, H., Schmid, M. & Hors, J. (1983) HLA-DR2 and IDD MOAD syndrome. *Lancet*, **ii**, 109.

Jordan, B. R., Lemonnier, F. A., Le Bouteiller, P., Malissen, M., Mishal, Z., Sodoyer, R., Delovitch, T. D., Strachan, T., Damotte, M., Nguyen, C., Layet, C., Dubreuil, J., van Agthoven, A. J., Trucy, J. & Caillol, D. (1983) Structure and expression of cloned HLA class I genes. In: *Progress in Immunology*, Vol. 5 (eds Y. Yamamura and T. Tada), p. 187. Academic Press.

Larhammar, D., Schenning, L., Gustafsson, K., Wiman, K., Claesson, L., Rask, L. & Peterson, P. A. (1982) Complete amino acid sequence of an HLA-DR antigen-like β chain as predicted from the nucleotide sequence: similarities with immunoglobulins and HLA-A, -B and -C antigens. *Proc. natn. Acad. Sci. U:S.A.* **79**, 3687.

Lemonnier, F. A., Dubreuil, P. C., Layet, C., Malissen, M., Bourel, D., Mercier, P., Jabobsen, B. K., Caillol, D. H., Svejgaard, A., Kourilsky, F. M. & Jordan, B. R. (1983) Transformation of the MLTK⁻ cells with purified HLA class I genes. II. Serologic characterization of HLA-A3 and Cw3 molecules. *Immunogenetics*, **18**, 65.

Marcadet, A., Fisher, A., Griscelli, L., Cohen, D. & Dausset, J. (1984) HLA genotyping using DNA probes in two cases of bare lymphocyte syndrome. (In preparation.)

Monson, J. P. & Boucher, B. J. (1983) HLA type and islet cell antibody status in family with (diabetes insipidus and mellitus, optic atrophy, and deafness) DIDMOAD syndrome. *Lancet*, **i**, 1286.

Owerbach, D., Lernmark, A., Platz, P., Ryder, L. P., Rask, L., Peterson, P. A. & Ludvigsson, J. (1983a) HLA-D region β-chain DNA endonuclease fragments differ between HLA identical healthy and insulin-dependent diabetic individuals. *Nature (Lond.)*, **303**, 815.

Owerbach, D., Lernmark, A., Rask, L., Peterson, P. A., Platz, P. & Svejgaard, A. (1983b) Detection of HLA-D/DR-related DNA polymorphism in HLA-D homozygous typing cells. *Proc. natn. Acad. Sci. U.S.A.* **80**, 3758.

Roux-Dosseto, M., Auffray, C., Lillie, J. W., Boss, J. M., Cohen, D., De Mars, R., Mawas, C., Seidman, J. G. & Strominger, J. L. (1983) Genetic mapping of a human classe II antigen β chain cDNA clone to the SB region of the HLA. *Proc. natn. Acad. Sci. U.S.A.* **80**, 6036.

Sood, A. K., Pereira, D. & Weissman, S. M. (1981) Isolation and partial nucleotide sequence of a cDNA clone for human histocompatibility antigen HLA-B by use of an oligodeoxynucleotide primer. *Proc. natn. Acad. Sci. U.S.A.* **78**, 616.

Trowsdale, J., Lee, J., Carey, J., Grosveld, F., Bodmer, J. & Bodmer, W. (1983) Sequences related to HLA-DR α chain on human chromosome 6: restriction enzyme polymorphism detected with DC α chain probes. *Proc. natn. Acad. Sci. U.S.A.* **80**, 1972.

Wake, C. T., Long, E. O. & Mach, B. (1982) Allelic polymorphism and complexity of the genes for HLA-DR β-chains direct analysis by DNA-DNA hybridization. *Nature (Lond.)*, **300**, 372.

Chapter 8
HLA-DRw6 and its impact on HLA-DR matching in renal transplantation

G. F. J. Hendriks, J. J. van Rood*, J. D'Amaro*,
G. G. Persijn, G. M. Th. Schreuder* & B. Cohen

*Eurotransplant Foundation and *Department of Immunohaematology and Blood Bank,
University Hospital, Rijnsburgerweg 10, 2333 AA Leiden, The Netherlands*

Summary. The effect of the presence or absence in the donor and recipient of HLA-DRw6 on the survival of first renal allografts was studied in 1792 recipients.

In 171 HLA-DRw6-positive recipients of one DR-mismatched allograft, graft survival at 1 year was significantly better when the donors were HLA-DRw6-positive than when they were HLA-DRw6-negative (80% *vs* 59%). In the group of 821 HLA-DRw6-negative recipients, graft survival at 1 year was also significantly better when the donors were HLA-DRw6-positive than when they were HLA-DRw6-negative for both one DR-mismatched (78% *vs* 67%) and two DR-mismatched (75% *vs* 66%) allografts.

Thus class II genes influence the homograft reaction in a very significant way, not only through the matching of donor and recipient, but also, at least for HLA-DRw6, via what is in all probability an Ir gene mechanism and by acting as activators or inducers of a suppressor cell circuit. We cannot say whether either of the two processes is due to the DRw6 gene coded for by the DR locus or the MBI gene coded for by the MB locus. It might be worthwhile to investigate whether the DR antigens interact primarily with helper T cells and the MB/MT antigens with suppressor/cytotoxic T cells.

Introduction

Since the early observations that a renal graft in HLA-matched donor–recipient sibling combinations had a prognosis far superior to that in HLA-mismatched sibling combinations, the question has been raised as to what extent these findings could be extrapolated to unrelated donor–recipient combinations. After more than 10 years of work and international collaboration, a provisional answer is available.

It has been shown in different studies that grafts which are identical for HLA-A, -B and -DR (or mismatched at most for one HLA-A or HLA-B antigen) survive extremely well. For all other match combinations, the extent of mismatching appears to have no effect on survival (Table 8.1). A patient file of 1500 or more should make it possible to provide at least 30–40% of the patients with a fully HLA-A, -B, -DR-matched, or at most one HLA-A or -B antigen-mismatched kidney graft. A large proportion of the patients can thus profit from HLA matching, but not all of them.

Table 8.1. Relation between the number of HLA-A, -B and -DR mismatches and graft survival

HLA-DR			0		1	2
HLA-A/B	0	1	2	3	0–3	0–3
1978	88*	86	—	—	60	61
1979	100	91	66	60	65	74
1980	90	86	61	50	72	68
1981	89	85	70	58	71	64
Total	91	86	67	55	68	6
(n)	(47)	(118)	(170)	(27)	(453)	(170) 6

* Actuarial life table estimates of probability (%) of graft survival at 1 year. In parentheses, number of patients at risk as given.

However, it is equally important that about two-thirds of the grafts which were mismatched for HLA-A, -B and -DR were functioning 1 year after transplantation. That may be due to an intrinsically reduced capability of these recipients to mount a homograft reaction. The investigations of that possibility is an important new development (Proceedings of the Second International Symposium on Immunological Monitoring of the Transplant Recipient/Eurotransplant Meeting, 1981).

Patients on haemodialysis (unlike healthy test persons) can be divided into low or high responders on the basis of their ability to respond to dinitrochlorobenzene (DNCB) in a skin test (Diamondopoulos, Hamilton & Briggs, 1979). Another variable that can be studied in such patients is an assay which measures the sensitivity of lymphocytes to prednisone in an antibody-dependent cytotoxicity (ADCC) test *in vitro* (Dumble *et al.*, 1983). The patients with a high sensitivity to prednisone had a very good graft survival, but those who were insensitive had poorer graft survival. Of all the variables which influence homograft reactivity, the factors which determine high or low DNCB skin test sensitivity, or prednisone sensitivity in an ADCC assay, may be the most important of all. Consequently, defining whether or not the recipient is a high responder before transplantation should be one of our first priorities. Apart from the functional tests described above, it may be possible to divide future recipients of renal allografts into high or low responder groups on the basis of immunogenetic data such as the ABO groups (Joysey *et al.*, 1973) and HLA-DR typing (Hendriks *et al.*, 1983b).

If the formation of antibodies against streptococcal, non-MHC, and HLA-DR antigens is taken as a reference point, DRw6-positive individuals are high responders (Lehner, 1982; Baldwin *et al.*, 1981; Hendriks *et al.*, 1983a). In agreement with this is the observation that HLA-DR matching is of great importance in DRw6-positive, and of far less importance in DRw6-negative recipients, as illustrated by the following analysis. The working hypothesis was that over the years in which HLA-DR matching was implemented, the results in DRw6-positive patients would have improved, while this would not be the case in DRw6-negative patients. The improvement would be gradual, because in the beginning HLA-DR typing could be performed mainly retrospectively after transplantation. Only recently it has become possible to type donors and recipients reliably before transplantation and to match them on the basis of HLA-DR. Our results have indeed shown that the 1 year graft survival in the DRw6-negative recipients remained the same over the years, while there was a striking and quite significant improvement of graft survival in the DRw6-positive recipients. Matching for DRw6 may, therefore, compensate for the high responsiveness of DRw6-positive recipients.

Table 8.2 summarizes the data of 1792 recipients. They are divided

Table 8.2. DRw6 and HLA-DR matching

DR match	Recipient	
	DRw6-pos.	DRw6-neg.
Compatible	82*	75
1 mismatch	68	69
2 mismatch	51	69
	$P = 0.003$	$P = 0.01$
	$n = 422$	$n = 1370$

* Actuarial life table estimates of probability (%) of graft survival at 1 year.

into two groups, those which are DRw6-positive and those which are DRw6-negative. There is a striking and significant effect of HLA-DR matching at 1 year after transplantation in the DRw6-positive group (a difference of 31% between the 0 and 2 DR mismatch classes), while the effect of HLA-DR matching in the DRw6-negative group is minimal (a difference of only 6% between 0 and 2 DR mismatch classes).

Naturally, the recipients will have received kidneys from DRw6-positive or from DRw6-negative donors. Table 8.3 illustrates how this influences graft survival. There are four divisions in Table 8.3. In the top left, donors and recipients are DRw6-positive ($n = 265$). One year after transplantation, graft survival was 82% and 77%, while the overall graft survival in the total group of 1792 recipients was only 67%. Thus, independent of the HLA-DR match, graft survival in this group was substantially better than the graft survival in the overall group. If the donor is DRw6-negative and the recipient DRw6-positive (top right, Table 8.3) a completely different picture emerges. Of course, there are no compatible grafts, and the one and two HLA-DR mismatches have a very poor graft survival (59% and 51% at 1 year, $n = 157$). If we combine the results of the DRw6-positive donors with those of the DRw6-negative

Table 8.3. DRw6 and HLA-DR matching

Recipient DRw6		Donor DRw6		
pos.		pos.		neg.
Compatible		82*		—
1 mismatch		77*		59*
2 mismatch		—		51*
(n) P	(265)	0·9	(157)	0·3
neg.		pos.		neg.
Compatible		—		75*
1 mismatch		78*		67*
2 mismatch		75*		66*
(n) P	(211)	0·4	(1159)	0·001
Total ($n = 1792$)			67*	

* Actuarial life table estimates of probability (%) of graft survival at 1 year.

ones, we reveal the origin of the striking effect of HLA-DR matching in the DRw6-positive recipients (Table 8.2). Although the results are significant, it is in effect an artefact which is caused by the DRw6 status of the donor.

If the donor is DRw6-positive and the recipient is DRw6-negative (bottom left, Table 8.3), the graft will be mismatched either for one or two HLA-DR antigens. However, independent of these mismatches, graft survival is good after 1 year and again better than the overall graft survival of the total group. Only in the group of patients in which both donor and recipient are DRw6-negative (bottom right, Table 8.3) do we observe a significantly beneficial effect of HLA-DR matching.

The DRw6 'gene effect' has been confirmed in some (Ting, personal communication; Hoitsma *et al.*, 1984; Soulilou & Bignon, 1983; UK Transplant, Bradley; Schmidt & Mayr, 1983), but not all centres (France Transplant, Betuel). The possible explanations for these discrepancies have been discussed extensively elsewhere (van Rood & Hendriks, 1984).

The clinical implications of these findings are self-evident. A DRw6-positive donor may be regarded as a universal donor, i.e. even very poor matches will show good graft survival.

If we design experiments to understand the mechanism which is responsible for this, we will be confronted with a problem which has been foremost in the minds of all HLA serologists, namely, the definition of DRw6. The definition of DRw6 is difficult, to say the least, and some workers have argued that it might not exist at all, a situation similar to the H-2 I-E null gene. Although there is biochemical evidence for its existence, nevertheless monospecific DRw6 antibodies are not available. As a consequence, DRw6 is defined mostly with antisera recognizing long or public specificities which are, at least in caucasoids, in very strong linkage disequilibrium with DRw6. The most important serum is anti-MB1 (MT1, LB-E12, DC1), which recognizes an antigen coded for by the MB locus closely linked to DR but separate from it. MB1 is in strong linkage disequilibrium not only with DRw6, but also with DR1, DR2 and DR10 (Schreuder *et al.*, 1983).

These facts logically lead to the question as to whether the 'DRw6-donor-effect' is due to DRw6 or to MB1 which is used to define it. We cannot answer this for the renal transplant data, although a recent analysis of the South-West German transplant group (Müller *et al.*, 1983) and a recent analysis by us is not incompatible with the assumption that the effect is related to MB1. Hard proof for this would need an *in vitro* system, which so far is lacking.

Data from Sasazuki *et al.* on suppressor T cell-dependent low responsiveness to streptococcal antigens associated with MT1 (Sasazuki *et al.*, 1983) and on the inhibition with the help of a monoclonal anti-MB1 antibody of the induction of cytotoxic T cells (Gorte *et al.*, 1982) could be in agreement with the hypothesis that antigens presented with DR activate primarily the helper circuit, and those which are presented with some MB/MT antigens the suppressor/cytotoxic circuit. Much of the above mentioned data and their discussion is reminiscent of what has been published about H-2 I-J (Tada, Taniguchi & David, 1976; Streilein & Klein, 1979). It remains to be verified to what extent DRw6 and I-J are really homologous.

Acknowledgments

This work was in part supported by the Dutch Foundation for Medical Research (FUNGO), which is subsidized by the Dutch Organization for the Advancement of Pure Research (ZWO), the J. A. Cohen Institute for Radiopathology and Radiation Protection (IRS), the Dutch Kidney Foundation, and the Eurotransplant Foundation.

We could not have done this analysis without the generous support of the physicians and the staff of all tissue-typing laboratories collaborating in Eurotransplant. We thank the staff of the Department of Immuno-haematology and Blood Bank for technical help, and Anne Pesant for preparing the manuscript.

References

Baldwin, W. M., Claas, F. H. J., van Es, L. A., van Rood, J. J., Paul, L. C. & Persijn, G. G. (1981) Renal graft rejection and the antigenic anatomy of human kidneys. In: *Transplantation and Clinical Immunology*, No. 12 (eds J. L. Touraine *et al.*), p. 140. Excerpta Medica, Amsterdam.

Diamondopoulos, A. A., Hamilton, D. N. H. & Briggs, J. D. (1979) A new predictive factor for the outcome of renal transplantation. In: *Proceedings of the European Dialysis and Transplantation Association, Istanbul, 1978* (eds B. H. B. Robinson and J. B. Hawkins), p. 283. Pitman Medical Publishing, Tunbridge Wells.

Dumble, L. J., MacDonald, I. M., Kincaid-Smith, P. & Clunie, G. J. A. (1983) Correlation between *in vitro* ADCC steroid resistance and renal allograft rejection. *Transplant. Proc.* **15**, 1145.

Gorte, G., Moretta, A., Cosulich, M. E., Ramarli, D. & Bergellesi, A. (1982) A monoclonal anti-DC1 antibody selectively inhibits the generation of effector T cells mediating specific cytolytic activity. *J. exp. Med.* **156**, 1539.

Hendriks, G. F. J., Claas, F. H. J., Persijn, G. G., Witvliet, M. D., Baldin, W. & Van Rood, J. J. (1983a) HLA-DRw6 positive recipients are high responders in renal transplantation. *Transplant. Proc.* **15**, 1136.

Hendriks, G. F. J., Schreuder, G. M. Th., Persijn, G. G., Cohen, B. & van Rood, J. J. (1983b) HLA-DRw6 and renal allograft rejection. *Br. med. J.* **286**, 85.

Hoitsma, H. J., Reekers, P., van Lier, H. J. J., van Rens, J. G. & Koene, R. A. P. (1984) HLA-DRw6 and treatment of acute rejection with anti-thymocyte globulin in renal transplantation. *Transplantation*, (in press).

Joysey, V. C., Roger, J. H., Evans, D. B. & Herbertson, B. M. (1973) Kidney graft survival and matching for HL-A and ABO antigens. *Nature (Lond.)*, **246**, 163.

Lehner, T. (1982) The relationship between human helper and suppressor factors to a streptococcal protein antigen. *J. Immunol.* **129**, 1936.

Müller, G. A., Müller, C., Bockhorn, H., Lenhard, V., Dreikorn, K., Fetta, R. F., Wilms, H., Fassbinder, W., Gumbel, B., Albert, F. W., Ewald, R. W., Goldmann, S., Sprenger-Klasen, I., Franz, H. E. & Wernet, P. (1983) HLA-DR-MT matching improves graft survival rate in cadaver kidney transplantation. *Klin. Wochenschr.* **61**, 17.

Proceedings of the Second International Symposium on Immunological Monitoring of the Transplant Recipient, in conjuction with the Eurotransplant Meeting; Noordwijkerhout/Leiden, September 18–20 1980 (1981) *Transplant. Proc.* **13**, 3.

Sasazuki, T., Nishimura, Y., Muto, M. & Ohta, N. (1983) HLA-linked genes controlling immune response and disease susceptibility. *Immunol. Rev.* **70**, 51.

Schmidt, G. F. J. & Mayr, W. R. (1983) HLA-DRw6 matching and primary renal graft failure due to rejection. *Lancet*, i, 1277.

Schreuder, G. M. Th., Parlevliet, J., Termijtelen, A. & van Rood, J. J. (1983) Reanalysis of the HLA-DRw6 complex. *Tiss. Antigens*, **21**, 62.

Singal, D. P., Mickey, M. R. & Terasaki, P. I. (1969) Serotyping for homotransplantation. XXIII. Analysis of kidney transplants from parental versus sibling donors. *Transplantation*, **7**, 246.

Soulillou, J. P. & Bignon, J. D. (1983) Poor kidney-graft survival in recipients with HLA-DRw6. *New Engl. J. Med.* **308**, 969.

Streilein, J. W. & Klein, J. (1979) Neonatal tolerance to K and D region alloantigens of H-2 complex: I-J region requirements. *Transplant. Proc.* **11**, 732.

Tada, T., Taniguchi, M. & David, C. S. (1976) Properties of the antigen-specific suppressive T-cell factor in the regulation of antibody response of the mouse. *J. exp. Med.* **144**, 713.

van Rood, J. J. & Hendriks, G. F. J. (1984) HLA matching, immune status and immunosuppression. In: *Transplantation and Clinical Immunology* (eds by J. L. Touraine *et al.*), (in press). Excerpta Medica, Amsterdam.

Chapter 9

Interaction between des-Tyr^1-γ-endorphins and HLA class I molecules: clinical relevance for the treatment of schizophrenia?

F. H. J. Claas*, R. Castelli-Visser*, B. M. de Jongh†,
J. J. van Rood*, W. M. A. Verhoeven‡, J. M. van Ree§
& D. de Wied§

*Department of Immunohaematology and Blood Bank, University Hospital Leiden,
Rijnsburgerweg 10, 2333 AA Leiden, † St. Lucas Hospital, Amsterdam, and
‡ Department of Psychiatry and § Rudolf Magnus Institute for Pharmacology,
State University of Utrecht, Utrecht, The Netherlands*

Summary. Pretreatment of lymphocytes from healthy donors with des-Tyr^1-γ-endorphin (DTγE) can inhibit the reaction between some HLA-alloantisera and their specific antigen.

A preferential inhibition of the reactivity of the sera was found against HLA-B15, Bw22, B13, A11, A10, Cw6 and Cw3, although other HLA antigens were partially inhibited.

A significant correlation was found between the *in vitro* inhibiting capacity of DTγE on the HLA antigen–antibody interaction and the HLA antigens of those schizophrenic patients who respond well to clinical treatment with γ-type endorphin.

Introduction

A variety of diseases are more common in individuals carrying certain antigens of the HLA system, the major histocompatibility complex (MHC) in man (Svejgaard, Platz & Ryder, 1983). Since regulation of immune responses is one of the main functions of the MHC, it is not surprising that many of these diseases have an immunological component in their pathogenesis. Nevertheless, non-immunological diseases have also been reported to be associated with HLA antigens. Such association could be due to chance, as is suggested for the localization of the gene for neuraminidase within the mouse H-2 complex (Klein, Figueroa & Klein, 1982). Another explanation is that the HLA molecules may be involved in ligand–receptor interactions, as postulated by Svejgaard & Ryder (1976).

Paranoid schizophrenia might be at first glance an example of such a non-immunological disease. It is associated with HLA-A9 and B5 (Ivanyi *et al.*, 1983). However, recently autoimmune mechanisms have been implicated in the aetiology of schizophrenia (Bergen *et al.*, 1980; Jancovics, Jakulic & Jorvat, 1980). The original hypothesis that schizophrenia is a metabolic disease might thus be only part of the pathogenesis of this disease.

After the discovery in pituitary and brain tissue of opioid peptides, endorphins, related to the pituitary hormone β-lipotropin, behavioural studies in rats have shown that the effects of γ-endorphin, β-endorphin [(βE)-1-17], and especially the non-opiate γ-endorphin fragments des-Tyr¹-γ-endorphin (DTγE, βE-2-17) and des-enkephalin γ-endorphin (DEγE, βE-6-17), correspond in certain aspects to those of classical neuropeptides (de Wied *et al.*, 1978). Subsequent clinical studies have shown that γ-type endorphins possess anti-psychotic properties in a number of schizophrenic patients (Verhoeven *et al.*, 1979; van Ree *et al.*, 1982). Genetic factors coded for within the HLA region may be associated with the response of patients to the treatment with γ-type endorphins, since HLA-B15 is increased in those patients who responded to treatment with γ-type endorphins and remained psychosis-free for a period of at least 6 months after treatment (van Ree *et al.*, 1982; de Jongh *et al.*, 1983). Receptor sites for opioids and endorphins have been demonstrated on peripheral blood lymphocytes (Hazum, Chang & Cuatrecasas, 1979; Mehrishi & Milles, 1983).

We now report that DTγE preferentially bind to certain HLA antigens, and that this *in vitro* interaction has a significant correlation with the *in vivo* clinical response to treatment with γ-type endorphins.

Materials and methods

We used a protocol very similar to the one developed for studies on the interaction between penicillin and certain HLA alloantigens (Claas *et al.*, 1982). Lymphocytes were prepared from heparinized blood of normal healthy donors by Ficoll-Hypaque density gradient centrifugation. An aliquot of these lymphocytes was incubated for 60 min at 4°C with graded concentrations of DTγE in phosphate-buffered saline (PBS). After washing with PBS, these lymphocytes were tested in a complement-dependent cytotoxicity assay against 120 well-defined HLA-A, -B, -C typing sera. In this assay 1 µl serum and 1 µl lymphocytes (2×10^6/ml) were incubated for 30 min at 4°C. After the addition of 5 µl rabbit complement, incubation was continued for another 60 min at 20°C. The percentage of dead cells were determined using eosin as a vital stain. Untreated lymphocytes from the same donors were tested in the same way, and the extent of inhibition (%) of the cytotoxicity was calculated by comparing the reactions of untreated and DTγE-treated lymphocytes.

Results

Isolated lymphocytes were preincubated with DTγE, and after washing, the binding of anti-HLA antibodies to their specific antigens was tested in a standard complement-dependent lymphocytotoxicity assay. The reactivity of the sera against pretreated cells was compared with that against untreated lymphocytes. The reactivity of antibodies against some HLA antigens was partially inhibited by DTγE, but other antibodies against HLA antigens showed no effect. The degree of inhibition was dependent on the concentration of DTγE used (Table 9.1). Maximal inhibition was found with 500 μg/ml, and further increasing the concentration of DTγE failed to increase the inhibition.

On the basis of the reactivity of 120 HLA alloantisera and lymphocytes of more than 30 healthy donors, a preferential inhibition of reactivity of the sera against HLA-B15 and HLA-Bw22 was found after

Table 9.1. Percentage inhibition of complement-dependent cytotoxicity after preincubation of the lymphocytes from a healthy volunteer (HLA: A2, Aw32, B15, B40) with graded concentrations of DTγE in phosphate-buffered saline

Molar concentration (DTγE; βE-2-17)		Serum 39991·5 (anti-B15)	Serum 33440·1 (anti-A2)
1 μg/ml	$6·0 \times 10^{-7}$	0	0
5 μg/ml	$3·0 \times 10^{-6}$	0	0
10 μg/ml	$6·0 \times 10^{-6}$	0	0
25 μg/ml	$1·5 \times 10^{-5}$	0	0
50 μg/ml	$3·0 \times 10^{-5}$	20	0
100 μg/ml	$6·0 \times 10^{-5}$	20	0
150 μg/ml	$9·0 \times 10^{-5}$	20	0
200 μg/ml	$1·2 \times 10^{-4}$	40	0
250 μg/ml	$1·5 \times 10^{-4}$	40	0
500 μg/ml	$3·0 \times 10^{-4}$	60	0
1000 μg/ml	$6·0 \times 10^{-4}$	60	0

preincubation of the cells with DTγE (Fig. 9.1). However, other HLA antigens were also partially blocked. Dilution experiments showed that these differences were not due to differences in the antibody titres of the sera.

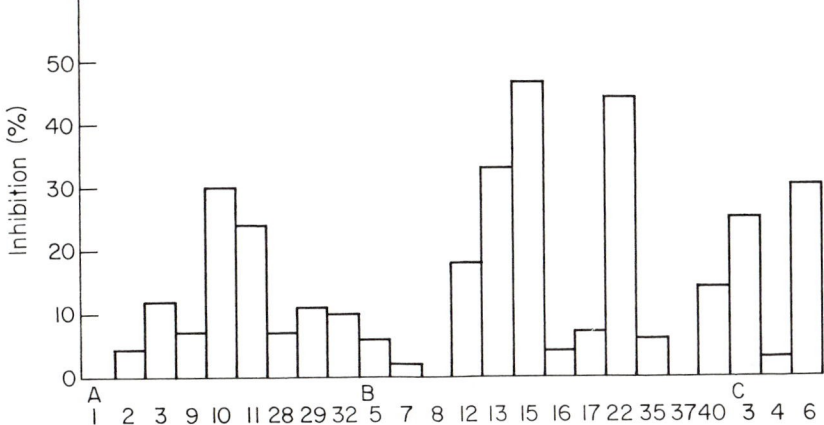

Fig. 9.1. The percentage lysis of HLA typing sera against the individual HLA-A, -B and -C antigens was determined both against untreated lymphocytes and lymphocytes from the same individual that had been incubated in a solution of DTγE (3×10^{-4} M).

The accumulated data of the reactions of at least two typing sera against the lymphocytes of at least three different individuals were collected and the percentage inhibition was calculated from the results obtained with untreated cells, as compared to cells treated with DTγE. This percentage is indicated on the vertical axis.

Using a similar approach, no inhibiting effect was found in the reaction of HLA-DR antisera with their corresponding antigens.

Next, the *in vitro* inhibitory capacity of DTγE was compared with the *in vivo* clinical response of patients to treatment with γ-type endorphin, as described previously (de Jongh *et al.*, 1983). The patients were divided into high and low responders on treatment with γ-type endorphins as assessed with the Brief Psychiatric Rating Scale (BPRS). When the HLA antigens of the high and low responders were compared, a relative risk (RR) among high responders as compared with low responders can be calculated for each individual HLA antigen. HLA-B15 showed a remarkable increase amongst the high responders (RR = 4·9) (de Jongh *et al.*, 1983). The association between the HLA class I antigens and the RR to become a high responder to the treatment with γ-type endorphin was not significant after correction for the number of antigens tested.

F. H. J. Claas et al.

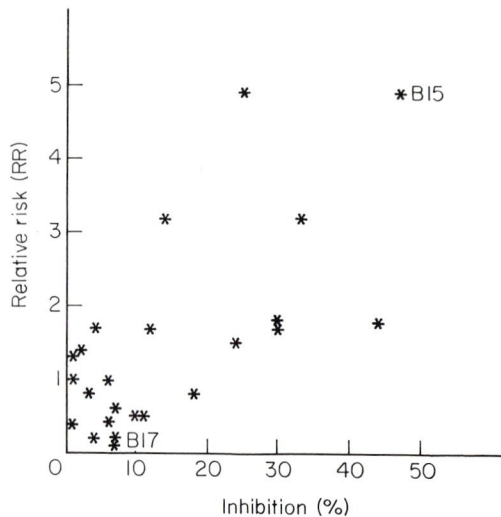

Fig. 9.2. Schizophrenic patients, treated with γ-type endorphin, were divided into high and low responders as assessed with the Brief Psychiatric Rating Scale (BPRS). By a comparison of the HLA phenotypes between the high and low responders, a relative risk (RR) to become a responder versus a non-responder was calculated for each individual HLA-A, -B and -C antigen (de Jongh *et al.*, 1983): i.e. HLA-B15 was remarkably increased among the high responders (RR = 4.9); HLA-B17 was increased among the low responders (RR = 0·1).

For every individual HLA-A, -B and -C antigen, the percentage inhibition found in the *in vitro* experiments (Fig. 9.1) was correlated with the RR of responses to clinical treatment with γ-type endorphins (correlation coefficient = 0·67; $P < 0.005$).

However, the number of antigens is not relevant when individual results are analysed between the *in vitro* inhibiting capacity of DTγE on HLA antigen–antibody interaction and the HLA antigens of those schizophrenic patients who respond to clinical treatment with γ-type endorphin. Figure 9.2 shows that there is a significant correlation between the *in vitro* inhibition by DTγE and the *in vivo* response to treatment with γ-type endorphins ($r = 0.67$, $P < 0.005$).

Discussion

The receptor/ligand theory of Svejgaard & Ryder (1976) is an attractive hypothesis especially for the endorphins, as recent data show that endorphins can affect the immune response. Alpha-endorphin can suppress the ability of mouse spleen cells to generate antibody responses both against thymus-dependent and thymus-independent antigens (Johnson *et al.*, 1982); β-endorphin can cause an increase in the proliferative response of rat spleen cells to concanavalin A (Gilman *et al.*, 1982) and can enhance the cytotoxicity by natural killer (NK) cells in man (Mathews *et al.*, 1983). With regard to schizophrenia, it has been reported that the neuroleptic chlorpromazine interferes with the binding of anti-HLA antibodies to some HLA antigens, especially to the HLA-A1 cross-reactive group (Smeraldi & Scorza-Smeraldi, 1976). A good response of schizophrenic patients to treatment with chlorpromazine was possibly associated with the presence of HLA-A1 (Smeraldi *et al.*, 1976). Similarly, the endogenous substance DTγE interferes with the binding of certain anti-HLA antibodies to their corresponding antigens. Especially those antigens, which are associated with a good clinical response to treatment with DTγE, have the highest affinity for DTγE. If confirmed, this kind of *in vitro* experiment may predict which patient will respond to treatment with neuroleptics or endogenous substances.

The interpretation of these results is uncertain. Binding studies with radioactive endorphin and membrane receptor precipitation experiments may reveal whether the HLA molecules are necessary and important for the binding of γ-endorphin to the cell. It may well be that the present results are due to binding of γ-endorphin to or near the HLA alloepitopes and that the specific endorphin receptor itself has only a loose association with the HLA molecules. This would be compatible with the finding that only up to 60% inhibition was found. Moreover, the expression of HLA antigens in brain tissue, where endorphins normally are found, is very weak (Berah, Hors & Dausset, 1970) and the beneficial effect of γ-endorphin therapy was found only in a limited number of patients by others (Emrich *et al.*, 1981).

The reason why an association is found between the treatment of schizophrenia and certain HLA antigens may be that HLA antigens function as (part of) the receptors for endogenous neuroactive substances. The existence of such receptor complexes is strongly suggested for insulin, as a close association on the cell membrane was found between insulin receptors and the major histocompatibility antigens (Simonsen & Olsson, 1983). Capping of all HLA class I antigens with a monoclonal antibody to an invariant heavy chain-MHC determinant nearly eliminated the binding of anti-insulin receptor antibodies. The same may hold for other endogenous substances. The present experiments suggest that epitopes detected by HLA alloantisera may play a role in the affinity of the receptor for its ligand.

Acknowledgments

This work was in part supported by the Dutch Foundation for Medical Research (FUNGO) which is subsidized by the Dutch Organization for the Advancement of Pure Research (ZWO), the J. A. Cohen Institute for Radiopathology and Radiation Protection (IRS).

References

Berah, M., Hors, J. & Dausset, J. (1970) A study of HL-A antigens in human organs. *Transplantation*, **9**, 185.

Bergen, J. T., Grinspoon, L., Pyle, H. M., Martinez, J. L. & Pennell, R. B. (1980) Immunologic studies in schizophrenic and control subjects. *Biol. Psychiat.* **15**, 369.

Claas, F. H. J., Runia-Van Nieuwkoop, R., van den Berge, W. & van Rood, J. J. (1982) Interaction of penicillin with HLA-A and -B antigens. *Human Immunol.* **5**, 83.

de Jongh, B. M., Verhoeven, W. M. A., van Ree, J. M., de Wied, D. & van Rood, J. J. (1983) HLA, and the response to treatment with γ-type endorphins in schizophrenia. *J. Immunogenet.* **9**, 381.

de Wied, D., Kovacs, G. L., Bohus, B., van Ree, J. M. & Greven, H. M. (1978) Neuroleptic activity of the neuropeptide β-LPH-62-77 (des-Tyr^1)-γ-endorphin (DTγE). *Eur. J. Pharmacol.* **49**, 427.

Emrich, H. M., Zaudig, M., Zerssen, D. V., Kissling, W., Oirlich, G. & Herz, A. (1981) Action of (Des-Tyr^1)-γ-endorphin in schizophrenia. *Mod. Prob. Pharmacopsychiat.* **17**, 279.

Gilman, S. C., Schwartz, J. M., Milner, R. J., Bloom, F. E. & Feldman, J. D. (1982) β-Endorphin enhances lymphocyte proliferative responses. *Proc. natn. Acad. Sci. U.S.A.* **79**, 4226.

Hazum, E., Chang, K. J. & Cuatrecasas, P. (1979) Specific non-opiate receptors for β-endorphin. *Science*, **205**, 1033.

Ivanyi, P., Droes, J., Schreuder, G. M. Th., d'Amaro, J. & van Rood (1983) A search for association of HLA antigens with paranoid schizophrenia: A9 appears as a possible marker. *Tiss. Antigens*, **22**, 186.

Jancovics, B. D., Jakulic, S. & Jorvat, J. (1980) Schizophrenia and other psychiatric diseases: evidence for neurotissue hypersensitivity. *Clin. exp. Immunol.* **40**, 515.

Johnson, H. M., Smith, E. M., Torres, B. A. & Blalock, J. E. (1982) Regulation of the *in vitro* antibody response by neuro-endocrine hormones. *Proc. natn. Acad. Sci. U.S.A.* **79**, 4171.

Klein, J., Figueroa, F. & Klein, D. (1982) H-2 haplotypes, genes and antigens: second listing. I. Non-H-2 loci on chromosome 17. *Immunogenetics*, **16**, 285.

Mathews, P. M., Froelich, C. J., Sibbit, W. L. & Bankhurst, A. D. (1983) Enhancement of natural cytotoxicity by β-endorphin. *J. Immunol.* **130**, 1658.

Mehrishi, J. N. & Milles, J. H. (1983) Opiate receptors on lymphocytes and platelets in man. *Clin. Immunol. Immunopathol.* **27**, 240.

Simonsen, M. & Olsson, L. (1983) Possible roles of compound membrane receptors in the immune system. *Ann. Immunol. (Inst. Pasteur)*, **134D**, 85.

Smeraldi, E., Bellodi, L., Sacchetti, E. & Cazullo, C. L. (1976) HLA The system and the clinical response to treatment with chlorpromazine. *Br. J. Psychiat.* **129**, 486.

Smeraldi, E. & Scorza-Smeraldi, R. (1976) Interference between anti-HLA antibodies and chlorpromazine. *Nature (Lond.)*, **260**, 532.

Svejgaard, A., Platz, P. & Ryder, L. P. (1983) HLA and disease 1982—a survey. *Immunol. Rev.* **70**, 193.

Svejgaard, A. & Ryder, L. P. (1976) Interaction of HLA molecules with non-immunological ligands as an explanation of HLA and disease associations. *Lancet*, **ii**, 547.

van Ree, J. M., Verhoeven, W. M. A., de Wied, D. & van Praag, H. M. (1982) The use of synthetic peptides γ-type endorphins in mentally ill patients. *Ann. N.Y. Acad. Sci.* **398**, 478.

Verhoeven, W. M. A., van Praag, H. M., van Ree, J. M. & de Wied, D. (1979) Improvement of schizophrenic patients treated with (des-Tyr^1)-γ-endorphin (DTγE). *Archs gen. Psychiat.* **36**, 294.

Index

Index